Dizziness, Hearing Loss, and Tinnitus:
The Essentials of Neurotology

Dizziness, Hearing Loss, and Tinnitus:
The Essentials of Neurotology

ROBERT W. BALOH, M.D.

Professor of Neurology and Surgery (Head and Neck)
Department of Neurology
Reed Neurological Research Center
University of California–Los Angeles
School of Medicine
Los Angeles, California

 F. A. DAVIS COMPANY · Philadelphia

NOTE:
As new information becomes available, recommended treatments and drug therapies undergo changes. The author and publisher have done everything possible to make this book accurate, up-to-date, and in accord with accepted standards at the time of publication. However, the reader is advised always to check product information (package inserts) for changes and new information before administering any drug.

Library of Congress Cataloging in Publication Data

Baloh, Robert W.
 Dizziness, hearing loss, and tinnitus.

 Bibliography: p.
 Includes index.
 1. Deafness. 2. Vertigo. 3. Tinnitus.
I. Title. II. Title: Essentials of neurotology. [DNLM: 1. Dizziness.
2. Hearing loss, Partial. 3. Tinnitus. 4. Ear—Innervation. 5. Ear—Physiology. WV 201 B195d]
RF290.B2   1984   617.8   83-15241
ISBN 0-8036-0581-1

To my wife Sandy

FOREWORD

Dizziness, Hearing Loss, and Tinnitus: The Essentials of Neurotology is a substantial contribution to the field of medical science dealing with neurotologic disease. The section on anatomy is quite detailed but is needed for a clear understanding of the clinical expressions of these disorders and for the interpretation of clinical test results. Also, the section on the physiology of the vestibular system is essential if the reader is to acquire a grasp of the manifestations of neurotologic disease. The section on pathology is well organized and supplemented with tables and charts that are useful in differential diagnosis. The text is well written. Grammar, sentence structure, and the more difficult concepts are clear and precise. I am particularly pleased to see the complete bibliography. Almost all statements are documented. The figures are clear and appropriate. It goes without saying that practitioners in the field of otolaryngology, neurology, and neurosurgery will want to have this book. The book should also be attractive to residents in otolaryngology, neurology, and neurosurgery. I believe that well informed and serious family practitioners and internists will also find this book to be useful.

Harold F. Schuknecht, M.D.

PREFACE

The purpose of this book is to present a concise, organized approach to evaluating patients with neurotologic symptoms (particularly dizziness, hearing loss, and tinnitus). The book is divided into three parts: Anatomy and Physiology, History and Examination, and Diagnosis and Treatment. In the first section, I briefly review clinically relevant anatomy and physiology to provide a framework for understanding the pathophysiology of vestibular and auditory symptoms. Part 2 outlines the important features in the patient's history and examination that determine the probable site of lesion. Finally, the section on diagnosis and treatment covers the key differential diagnostic points that help the clinician decide on the cause of the patient's problem and how to treat it. I included separate chapters on the symptomatic treatment of dizziness and tinnitus, because one is often faced with treating these symptoms on an empirical basis.

It is my hope that this book will be useful to all physicians who deal with patients complaining of dizziness, hearing loss, and/or tinnitus. It can serve as an introduction to neurotology for students and resident physicians and as a practical reference source for practicing clinicians. I have attempted to maintain a balanced presentation of otologic and neurologic disorders, because I strongly believe that one cannot effectively evaluate neurotologic problems without understanding both the peripheral and central aspects of these disorders. Since my background is primarily in neurology, however, this book is a neurologist's view of neurotology.

RWB

ACKNOWLEDGMENTS

One needs a great deal of help and advice from colleagues to formulate ideas for a book such as this. I have been extremely fortunate to have two exceptional co-workers since I joined the neurology staff at UCLA in the early 1970s. Dr. Vicente Honrubia in otolaryngology and Dr. Robert D. Yee in ophthalmology share in all my accomplishments because we have always worked as a team. Two other key members of our research team are Susan Sakala and Laurn Langhofer. I am grateful for the constant support of Drs. Augustus Rose, Richard D. Walter, and Paul H. Ward, which has allowed me to concentrate my efforts in the area of neurotology. Drs. Harold Schuknecht, Paul Brownstone, and Elliot Abemayor provided helpful comments and suggestions after reviewing the manuscript. Finally, I want to acknowledge the long-standing support for my work by the National Institutes of Health.

RWB

CONTENTS

xiii

PART 2   HISTORY AND EXAMINATION

PART 1
ANATOMY AND PHYSIOLOGY

1

THE MIDDLE EAR

COMPONENTS

DEVELOPMENT

BOUNDARIES OF THE TYMPANIC CAVITY

EUSTACHIAN TUBE

TYMPANIC MEMBRANE

THE OSSICULAR CHAIN

FACIAL NERVE

COMPONENTS

The middle ear consists of a series of irregular, pneumatic chambers within the temporal bone.[1] Three main chambers are routinely identified: the tympanic cavity, the mastoid antrum, and the eustachian tube (Fig. 1). The centrally located tympanic cavity, situated between the external and internal ear, is traversed by a chain of small bones that transmit vibrations from the tympanic membrane to the labyrinth. The tympanic cavity can be subdivided into a lower part corresponding in vertical extent to the tympanic membrane and an upper region extending above the upper border of the tympanic membrane, known as the epitympanic recess. The mastoid antrum, an irregular, bean-shaped cavity, communicates with the posterior epitympanic recess by an aperture, the aditus ad antrum. Many of the pneumatized spaces of the mastoid open directly into the antrum. Finally, the tympanic cavity communicates directly with the pharynx via the elongated eustachian tube.

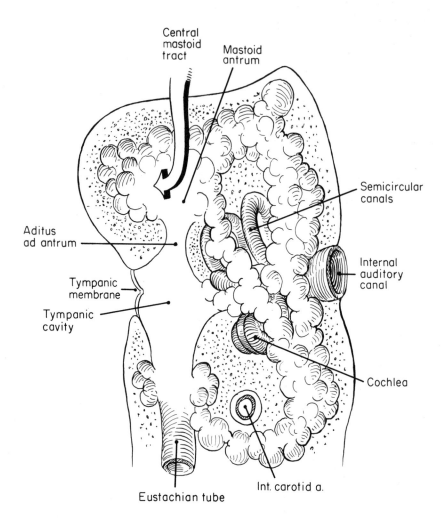

Central mastoid tract

Mastoid antrum

Semicircular canals

Aditus ad antrum

Internal auditory canal

Tympanic membrane

Tympanic cavity

Cochlea

Int. carotid a.

Eustachian tube

FIGURE 1. Schematic drawing of intercommunicating air cell system within the temporal bone. (Adapted from Schuknecht, HF: *Pathology of the Ear.* Harvard University Press, Cambridge, MA, 1974).

DEVELOPMENT

In the embryo the middle ear develops from a pouch of the primitive gut, the first pharyngeal pouch.[1,2] As this pouch of entodermal origin moves towards the developing temporal bone, the mesenchymal tissue that fills the middle ear of the fetus recedes. Ciliated epithelium from the primitive gut covers the eustachian tube, tympanic cavity, and mastoid, forming an endless variety of small cavities in a process known as pneumatization (see Fig. 1). The degree of pneumatization of the human temporal bone varies greatly, depending on hereditary factors, nutrition, and the adequacy of ventilation via the eustachian tube.[3] Each pneumatized space is usually in free communication with all other pneumatized spaces. Passageways that interconnect these air cells (e.g., the central mastoid tract shown by the arrow in Fig. 1) serve as routes for infection to follow as it spreads from the middle ear through the temporal bone.[3,4]

BOUNDARIES OF THE TYMPANIC CAVITY

The *lateral wall* of the tympanic cavity consists mainly of the tympanic membrane, together with the small rim of temporal bone to which it is attached. Superiorly, the lateral wall of the epitympanic recess is formed by the scutum, a plate of bone belonging to the squamous part of the temporal bone. The *medial wall* of the tympanic cavity is irregular owing to several structures bulging from the inner ear: the promontory of the basal turn of the cochlea and the prominences of the facial canal and horizontal semicircular canal (Fig. 2). The round window is located inferior and posterior to the promontory of the cochlea. This membrane seals the fluid in the scala tympani of the cochlea from the tympanic cavity. Posterior to the promontory is a smooth projection, the support of the promontory or the subiculum, which forms the inferior border of a deep depression known as the tympanic sinus. The oval window is located just above the promontory. It is closed by the stapes and the annular ligament.

The *anterior or carotid wall* of the tympanic cavity contains, from above to below, the insertion of the tensor tympani muscle, the orifice of the eustachian tube, and a thin bony wall covered with air cells separating the tympanic cavity from the carotid canal. The *posterior or mastoid wall* contains the aditus ad antrum, an aperture transmitting the tendon of the stapedius muscle, a foramen by which the chorda tympani nerve enters the middle ear, and a fossa where the posterior ligament of the incus is attached.

The *roof* of the tympanic cavity is formed by the tegmen tympani, a thin plate of bone separating the epitympanic recess of the middle ear from the middle cranial fossa. The *floor* is very narrow transversely, being closely related to the fossa of the internal jugular vein. It is irregular owing to the large number of air cells, and near the back there is a stylomastoid prominence corresponding to the root of the styloid process.

EUSTACHIAN TUBE

The eustachian tube connects the tympanic cavity with the nasopharynx, providing ventilation of the tympanic cavity and the adjacent pneumatized cavities of the temporal bone (see Figs. 1 and 2). The tubal orifice at the nasopharynx is normally closed, but during deglutition it opens owing to contraction of palate muscles that attach to the cartilage and elastic ligaments around the opening. The tensor veli palati, the levator veli palati and the salpingopharyngeus muscles simultaneously contract during the act of swallowing or yawning, causing

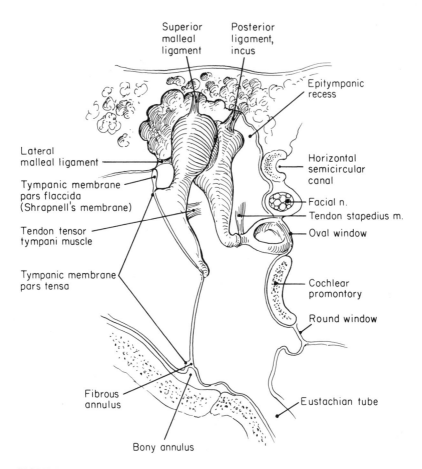

FIGURE 2. Cross section of the tympanic membrane and tympanic cavity.

rotation and forceful pulling apart of the lateral and medial laminae of the eustachian tube cartilage. The tensor veli palati, the most important of these muscles, is supplied by the mandibular division of the trigeminal nerve.

Failure of the eustachian tube to open during deglutition results in negative pressure in the pneumatized spaces of the temporal bone as a consequence of gases being absorbed into the blood stream. Improper opening of the eustachian tube may be due to an inflammatory reaction of the lining membrane such as occurs with infection or allergies of the upper respiratory tract. Other factors producing narrowing of the lumen include hyperplasia of lymphoid tissue, muscle weakness, neoplasia, and developmental anomalies such as those associated with cleft palate. Inadequate ventilative function of the eustachian tube in early life may inhibit pneumatization of the temporal bone and lead to chronic

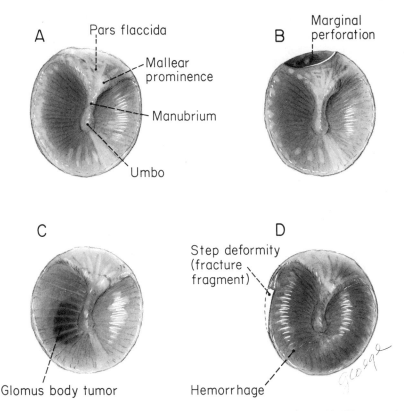

A — Pars flaccida, Mallear prominence, Manubrium, Umbo

B — Marginal perforation

C — Glomus body tumor

D — Step deformity (fracture fragment), Hemorrhage

FIGURE 3. View of the tympanic membrane from the external ear canal in (A) a normal subject, and in patients with (B) a superior marginal perforation and cholesteatoma, (C) a tympanic glomus body tumor, and (D) a step deformity caused by a longitudinal temporal bone fracture. (From Baloh, RW and Honrubia, V: *Clinical Neurophysiology of the Vestibular System.* FA Davis, Philadelphia, 1979, with permission).

middle ear infections. Eustachian tube dysfunction is probably a major factor in the etiology of seromucinous otitis media.[5]

TYMPANIC MEMBRANE

The tympanic membrane consists of three layers: an inner mucosal layer, a middle fibrous layer, and an external epidermal layer. It is conical in shape with a diameter ranging from 8.5 to 10 mm. From the external canal the tympanic membrane appears as a thin semitransparent disc that normally has a glistening pearly-gray color (Fig. 3A). It is concave on its external surface, as if under traction from the manubrium of the malleus. The mallear stria (the manubrium shining through the tympanic membrane) passes from slightly inferior and posterior of the center (umbo) toward the superior margin of the tympanic membrane. Near the superior margin the mallear prominence is formed by the lateral process of the malleus. From the mallear prominence, two folds stretch to the tympanic sulcus of the temporal bone enclosing the triangular area of the pars flaccida, or Shrapnell's membrane. Rupture of the membrane at this site is commonly associated with invasion of the middle ear by keratinizing squamous epithelium from the external ear canal (Fig. 3B). This keratoma, or cholesteatoma, usually develops in the epitympanic space, from which it may extend posteriorly into the antrum and the central mastoid tract, inferiorly into the middle ear, where it may erode the ossicles and bony labyrinth, and superiorly into the intracranial cavity, producing central nervous system symptoms and signs.[3] Because of its semitransparency, lesions within the tympanic cavity often can be seen through the tympanic membrane (e.g., Figs. 3C and 3D).

THE OSSICULAR CHAIN

The ossicles provide an interface for transmitting to the inner ear changes in atmospheric pressure produced by sound waves. The long process of the malleus, the manubrium, is attached like the radius of a circle to the inner side of the tympanic membrane in a supero-anterior direction (see Fig. 2). Superiorly, the head of the malleus is bound to the incus, forming the incudomalleal articulation, a type of diarthric joint. The long process of the incus directed down and anteriorly is connected to the stapes, the smallest of the three middle ear ossicles. The footplate of the stapes articulates with the walls of the vestibule at the oval window, to which it is attached by a ring of ligaments. The dimensions of the window are 1.2 by 3 mm, with a total area that is one-seventeenth that of the tympanic membrane. Sound-induced displacements of the tympanic membrane and its attached manubrium are transmitted through the medial arm of the assembly of middle ear bones acting as a lever to the inner ear; in this fashion the middle ear functions as a mechanical transformer. Additional amplification is produced as the force applied over the surface of the tympanic membrane is funneled into the smaller area of the oval window. The middle ear compensates for the loss of energy that would occur if sound were directly transmitted from air to the fluids of the inner ear. Without the middle ear structures, approximately 99.9 percent of the sound energy would be lost during this transmission.[6]

The ossicles are suspended by several ligaments and are dynamically controlled by the action of two muscles (see Fig. 2). The tensor tympani, innervated by a branch of the trigeminal nerve, is connected by a tendon into the upper part of the manubrium. Coursing in a lateral direction from the anterior part of the medial wall of the tympanic cavity, this muscle draws the manubrium medially, tensing the tympanic membrane. The stapedius muscle, innervated by the facial nerve, is attached to the posterior wall of the tympanic cavity and is directed anteriorly to anchor in the upper part of the stapes. Its contraction hinders the transmission of sound to the inner ear.

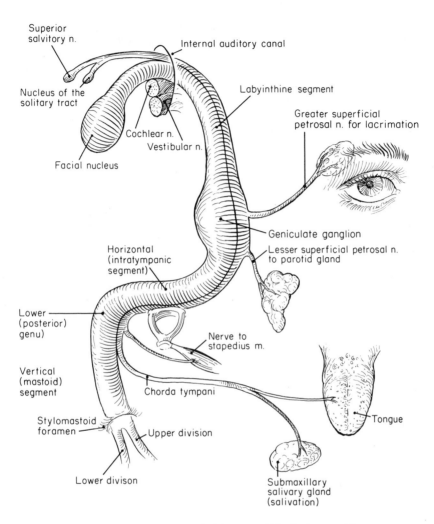

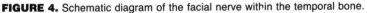

FIGURE 4. Schematic diagram of the facial nerve within the temporal bone.

FACIAL NERVE

The facial nerve arises at the inferior border of the pons and proceeds to the internal auditory canal on the superior surface of the cochlear nerve.[7] Within the temporal bone four portions of the facial nerve can be classified: (1) the canal segment, (2) the labyrinthine segment, (3) the tympanic (horizontal) segment, and (4) the mastoid (vertical) segment (Fig. 4). The canal segment runs in close company with the vestibular and cochlear division of the eighth nerve, while in its remaining segments the facial nerve lies separately within a bony canal, the facial, or fallopian canal. The labyrinthine segment runs at nearly a right angle to the petrous pyramid superior to the cochlea and vestibule to reach the geniculate ganglion. At the geniculate ganglion the nerve takes a sharp turn posteriorly, marking the beginning of the tympanic segment. The tympanic segment passes along the medial wall of the tympanic cavity superior to the oval window and inferior to the horizontal semicircular canal. At the sinus tympani the nerve bends inferiorly, marking the beginning of the mastoid segment.

Four branches of the facial nerve lie within the temporal bone: the greater and lesser superficial petrosal nerves arising from the geniculate ganglion, the nerve to the stapedius muscle arising from the mastoid segment as it crosses the middle ear, and the chorda tympani leaving the facial nerve approximately 5 mm above the stylomastoid foramen (see Fig. 4). The greater superficial petrosal nerve is composed of parasympathetic efferent fibers originating in the superior salivatory nucleus for innervation of the lacrimal glands and seromucinous glands of the nasal cavity, and afferent cutaneous sensory fibers from parts of the external canal, tympanic membrane and middle ear destined for the nucleus of the solitary tract. The lesser superficial petrosal nerve contains parasympathetic efferent fibers for the salivary glands. The nerve to the stapedius muscle and the main facial nerve trunk are motor nerves originating from the facial nucleus in the caudal pons. The chorda tympani, like the greater superficial petrosal, is a mixed nerve containing parasympathetic efferent fibers from the superior salivatory nucleus destined for the submaxillary glands, and afferent taste fibers from the anterior two-thirds of the tongue ending in the nucleus of the solitary tract.

Knowledge of the structure and function of each division of the facial nerve allows the clinician to localize lesions affecting the nerve within the temporal bone. Lesions in the internal auditory canal commonly involve both the seventh and eighth cranial nerves. Lesions of the labyrinthine segment of the facial nerve above the geniculate ganglion impair ipsilateral (1) lacrimation, (2) salivation, (3) stapedius reflex activity, (4) taste on the anterior two-thirds of the tongue, and (5) facial muscular strength. A lesion of the tympanic segment central to the nerve of the stapedius muscles affects only (3), (4) and (5) of the above and a lesion of the mastoid segment before the origin of the chorda tympani affects only (4) and (5). Finally, a lesion at the stylomastoid foramen causes only ipsilateral facial muscle weakness or paralysis.

REFERENCES

1. ANSON, BJ, AND DONALDSON, JA: *Surgical Anatomy of the Temporal Bone, ed 3.* WB Saunders, Philadelphia, 1981.

2. PEARSON, AA: *The Development of the Ear: A Manual.* Rochester, MN. American Academy of Ophthalmology and Otolaryngology, 1967.

3. SCHUKNECHT, HF: *Pathology of the Ear.* Harvard University Press, Cambridge, MA, 1974.

4. ALLAM, A: *Pneumatization of the temporal bone.* Ann Otol Rhinol Laryngol 78:49, 1969.

5. BLUESTONE, C, BEERY, Q, AND ANDRUS, W: *Mechanics of eustachian tube as it influences susceptibility to and persistence of middle ear effusions in children.* Ann Otol Rhinol Laryngol (Suppl) 83 (11):27, 1974.

6. WEVER, E, AND LAWRENCE, M: *Physiological Acoustics.* Princeton University Press, Princeton, 1954.

7. CARPENTER, MB: *Core Text of Neuroanatomy, ed 7.* Williams & Wilkins, Baltimore, 1976.

2

THE INNER EAR

PHYLOGENY OF THE LABYRINTH

The earliest gravity receptor organ, the statocyst, appeared more than 600 million years ago, in the late Precambrian era.[1] Beginning with primitive jellyfish, the statocyst allowed the animal to orient itself in relation to the horizon by sensing the direction of the gravitational force of the earth. The statocyst is a fluid-filled invagination, or sac, containing a calcinous particle, the statolith, or multiple particles, the statoconia, of density greater than the fluid. Attracted by gravity, the particles rest their weight differentially over special cells in the wall of the cyst. The direction of the force on the underlying sensory cells therefore depends on the position of the animal in space.

A continuous increment in anatomic complexity occurs in evolution of the simple statocyst to the labyrinth of higher animals.[2] In primitive fish (cyclostomes) the statocyst cavity, previously open to the outside, is closed and filled by an endogenous secretion (endolymph). Two surviving cyclostomes, the hagfish and lamprey, demonstrate an important step in the phylogenetic development of the vestibular labyrinth. In the hagfish, a simple circular tube is interrupted anteriorly and posteriorly by bulbous enlargements, the ampullae, each containing a primitive crista. Between the ampullae in an intercommunicating channel lies the macule communis, the forerunner of the utricular and saccular macules. The labyrinth of the lamprey is more complex, consisting of an anterior and posterior canal communicating with a bilobulated sac containing separate utricular and saccular macules.

The predecessor of the cochlea appears after the development of a membranous labyrinth that is divided into two cavities.[3] In the inferior of the two cavities (the saccule), two new receptor areas develop, the lagenar macule and the basilar papilla. The basilar papilla is small compared with the lagena in amphibia. In reptiles, a gradual enlargement of the basilar papilla occurs, so that in the crocodile the recess of the basilar papilla forms a long tube, the cochlear duct. The lagena in crocodiles and birds is displaced into a widened blind sac forming the end of the cochlear duct. The curvature of the cochlear duct is slight in birds, but is much more pronounced in mammals, where a varying number of coils form a complete cochlea. The basilar membrane first appears in the reptilian stage of evolution. The sensory epithelium of the basilar membrane forms the basilar papilla in birds, and the organ of Corti in mammals.

DEVELOPMENT OF THE LABYRINTH

In the embryo the membranous labyrinth begins as ectodermal thickenings, the otic placodes, on each side of the rhombencephalon (Fig. 5).[4] The primitive otocyst forms by invagination of the otic placode, which becomes the inner layer of the membranous labyrinth. Three primary components develop through infolding of the walls of the otocyst: (1) the endolymphatic duct and sac, (2) the utricle and semicircular canals, and (3) the saccule and cochlear duct. The walls of the membranous labyrinth consist of an inner layer of ectodermal origin and an outer layer of mesodermal origin, separated by a basement membrane. Regions of the inner layer subsequently develop into the specialized sensory organs.

It is helpful to know the interrelationships and timing of the development of the different inner ear structures, since congenital developmental defects can occur at each stage of development. The inner ear begins to develop approximately three weeks after conception, with the appearance of the placodes. The placode rapidly forms the otocyst, and invagination within the vesicular wall divides it into vestibular and cochlear components (Fig. 5A–C). Concurrent with placode-otocyst development, the stato-acousticofacial ganglion forms from the neural crest at the end of the third week. The otocyst develops into the vestibular duct, from which an anteroinferior cochlear diverticulum develops (Fig. 5D).

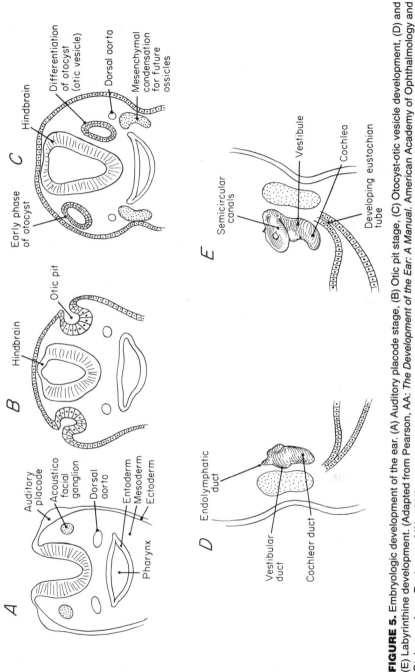

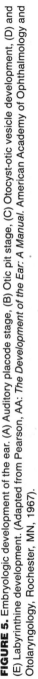

FIGURE 5. Embryologic development of the ear. (A) Auditory placode stage, (B) Otic pit stage, (C) Otocyst-otic vesicle development, (D) and (E) Labyrinthine development. (Adapted from Pearson, AA: *The Development of the Ear: A Manual*. American Academy of Ophthalmology and Otolaryngology, Rochester, MN, 1967).

By the end of the fourth week of development the vestibular duct differentiates into the three semicircular canals as the cochlear duct begins to develop from its inferior, saccular portion (Fig. 5E). The cochlear turns begin to form by the sixth to seventh week with completion of two and one-half turns by the eighth week. By the fifth month, the primitive organ of Corti is formed within the cochlear duct. The stato-acousticofacial ganglion divides into a superior portion that sends fibers to the utricle and ampullae of the anterior and horizontal semicircular canals, and an inferior portion that sends fibers to the saccule and ampulla of the posterior semicircular canal. The remainder of the acoustic ganglion becomes the spiral ganglion of the cochlea.

FLUID DYNAMICS OF THE INNER EAR

The bony labyrinth is a series of hollow channels within the petrous portion of the temporal bone (Fig. 6). It consists of an anterior cochlear part, a posterior vestibular part, and a central chamber, the vestibule. Medial to the bony labyrinth is the internal auditory canal, a cul-de-sac housing the VII and VIII cranial nerves and internal auditory artery. The aperture on the cranial side is located at approximately the center of the posterior face of the pyramid of the temporal bone. Two other important orifices are in this vicinity. Halfway between the opening of the internal auditory canal and the sigmoid sinus, the slit-like aperture of the vestibular aqueduct contains the endolymphatic sac, a structure important in the exchange of endolymph. The second opening is that of the cochlear aqueduct, at the same level as the internal auditory canal, but on the inferior side of the pyramid. The labyrinthine opening of this channel is located in the scala tympani, providing a connection between the subarachnoid and the perilymphatic spaces. The membranous labyrinth is enclosed within the channels of the bony labyrinth. A space containing perilymphatic fluid, a supportive network of connective tissue and blood vessels, lies between the periosteum of the bony labyrinth and the membranous labyrinth; the spaces within the membranous labyrinth contain endolymphatic fluid.

Perilymph is primarily formed by filtration from blood vessels in the inner ear.[5,6] As indicated above, perilymph communicates with the cerebrospinal fluid (CSF) through the cochlear aqueduct, a narrow channel 3 to 4 mm long, with its inner ear opening at the base of the scala tympani (see Fig. 6). In most instances this channel is filled by a loose net of fibrous tissue continuous with the arachnoid. The size of the bony canal varies from individual to individual. Infection and blood within the CSF can make their way to the inner ear via the cochlear aqueduct.

The most likely site for production of endolymph is the secretory cells in the stria vascularis of the cochlea and the dark cells of the vestibular labyrinth.[7] Resorption of endolymph is generally agreed to take place in the endolymphatic sac (see Fig. 6). Dye and pigment injected experimentally into the cochlea of animals accumulate in the endolymphatic sac; electron microscopic studies of the lining membrane of the sac reveal active pinocytotic activity.[6,8] Destruction of the epithelium lining the sac, or occlusion of the duct, results in an increase of

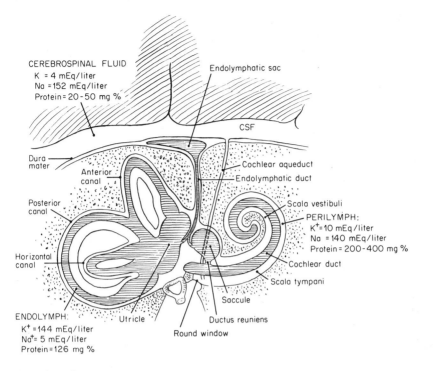

CEREBROSPINAL FLUID
K = 4 mEq/liter
Na =152 mEq/liter
Protein= 20-50 mg %

Endolymphatic sac

CSF

Dura mater

Anterior canal

Posterior canal

Horizontal canal

ENDOLYMPH:
K⁺ =144 mEq/liter
Na⁺= 5 mEq/liter
Protein=126 mg %

Utricle

Cochlear aqueduct

Endolymphatic duct

Scala vestibuli

PERILYMPH:
K⁺=10 mEq/liter
Na =140 mEq/liter
Protein= 200-400 mg %

Cochlear duct

Scala tympani

Saccule

Ductus reuniens

Round window

FIGURE 6. Fluid compartments of the inner ear.

endolymphatic volume in experimental animals.[9,10] The first change is an expansion of cochlear and saccular membranes that may completely fill the perilymphatic spaces. The anatomic changes resulting from this experiment are comparable to those found in the temporal bones of patients with Meniere's syndrome (either idiopathic or secondary to known inflammatory disease) (see Fig. 59).

The chemical composition of the fluids filling the inner ear is similar to that of the extracellular and intracellular fluids throughout the body. The endolymphatic system contains intracellular-like fluids with a high potassium and low sodium concentration, while the perilymphatic fluid resembles the extracellular fluids, having a low potassium and high sodium concentration (see Fig. 6).[11] The endolymphatic sac has a much higher protein content than the endolymphatic space, consistent with its role in the resorption of endolymph. The electrolyte composition of the endolymph and perilymph is critical for normal functioning of the sensory organs bathed in fluid. Ruptures of the membranous labyrinth in experimental animals cause destruction of the sensory and neural structures at the site of the endolymph-perilymph fistula.[12] Spontaneous ruptures of the membranous labyrinth may be the cause of episodic symptoms in patients with Meniere's syndrome. With the rupture, potassium leaks from the endolymph to perilymph, inhibiting the bioelectric activity of the cochlear and vestibular hair cells. The potassium is then slowly cleared from the perilymph and labyrinthine function returns to normal within 2 to 3 hours (i.e., a typical duration of an attack in Meniere's syndrome).

BLOOD SUPPLY OF THE INNER EAR

The artery that supplies the membranous labyrinth and its neural structures is a branch of an intracranial vessel and does not communicate with arteries in the otic capsule and middle ear.[6,13] This vessel, the internal auditory artery, usually originates from the anterior inferior cerebellar artery, but exceptionally it arises directly from the basilar artery or some of its branches (Fig. 7; also see Figs. 53 and 54). As it enters the temporal bone it forms branches that irrigate the ganglion cells, nerves, dura, and arachnoidal membranes in the internal auditory canal. Shortly after entering the inner ear, the labyrinthine artery divides into two main branches, the common cochlear artery and the anterior vestibular artery. Because the arteries course independently, occlusion of one branch can result in selective damage to one part of the labyrinth. The common cochlear artery forms two branches, the posterior vestibular artery and the main cochlear artery. The latter enters the central canal of the cochlea, where it generates the radiating arterioles forming a plexus within the cochlea irrigating the spiral ganglion, the structures in the basilar membrane and the stria vascularis. The posterior vestibular artery, a branch from the common cochlear artery, is the source of blood supply to the inferior part of the saccule and the ampulla of the posterior semicircular canal. The other primary branch of the labyrinthine artery, the anterior vestibular branch, provides irrigation to the utricle and ampulla of the anterior and horizontal semicircular canals, as well as some blood to a small portion of the saccule.

Interruption of the blood supply in the internal auditory artery or any of its branches seriously impairs the function of the inner ear, since the labyrinthine arteries do not anastomose with any other major arterial branch.[6,14] Within 15 seconds of blood flow interruption, the auditory nerve fibers become inexcitable, and the receptor and resting potentials in the ear abruptly diminish. If the interruption lasts for a prolonged period of time the changes are irreversible; loss of function is followed by degenerative changes wherein ganglion cells and sensory cells undergo autolysis and new bone growth fills the ear cavity.

THE HAIR CELL

The basic element of the inner ear that transduces the mechanical forces associated with sound and head acceleration to nerve action potentials is the hair cell.[15] Two types of hair cells occur in birds and mammals (Fig. 8). Type II cells are cylindrical, with multiple nerve terminals at their base, while type I cells are globular or flask-shaped, with a single large chalice-like nerve terminal surrounding the base. A bundle of nonmobile stereocilia protrudes from the cuticular plate on the apical end of each receptor cell. The height of the stereocilia

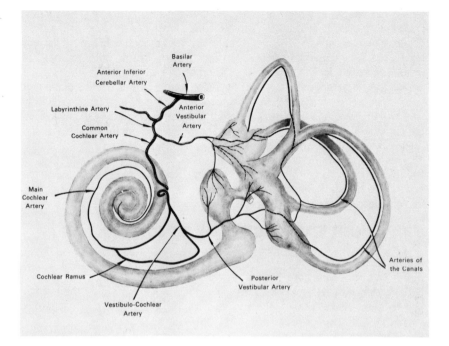

FIGURE 7. Arterial supply to the inner ear. (From Schuknecht, HF: *Pathology of the Ear.* Harvard University Press, Cambridge, MA, 1974, with permission).

increases stepwise from one side to the other, and next to the tallest stereocilia a thicker, longer hair, the kinocilium, protrudes from the cell's cytoplasm through a segment of cell membrane lacking the cuticular plate. Hair cells in the cochlea have only a rudimentary kinocilium.

The adequate stimulus for hair cell activation is a force acting parallel to the top of the cell, resulting in bending of the hairs (a shearing force).[16] A force applied perpendicular to the cell surface (a compressional force) is ineffective in stimulating the hair cell. The stimulus is maximal when the force is directed along an axis that bisects the bundle of stereocilia and goes through the kinocilium. Deflection of the hairs toward the kinocilium decreases the resting membrane potential of the sensory cells (depolarization). Bending in the opposite direction produces the reverse effect (hyperpolarization).

Most of the basic information regarding the physiologic properties of hair cells and their afferent nerves has been obtained through a study of hair cell systems in nonmammalian species.[17] Analysis of the lateral line organs of fish and amphibians has been particularly useful. These organs consist of groups of hair cells, the neuromasts, aligned in longitudinal rows on the side of the animal's body and head. A free-standing gelatinous cupula covering the hairs transmits the force associated with water displacement into hair cell deflection that in turn results in a change in firing rate of the afferent nerve. The afferen nerves from lateral line organs generate continuous spontaneous activity. This observation has subsequently been confirmed in all other hair cell systems, and represents a fundamental discovery in sensory physiology. While the mechanism responsible for the spontaneous firing of action potentials in the afferent nerves has not been identified, depolarization and hyperpolarization of the hair cells' membrane potential result in a modulation of this spontaneous activity (see Fig. 8). Bending of the hairs toward the kinocilium results in an increase of the spontaneous firing rate, and bending of the hairs away from the kinocilium results in a decrease. The spontaneous firing rate varies among different animal species and among different sensory receptors. It is thought to be greatest in the afferent neurons of the semicircular canals of mammals (up to 90 spikes per second), and lowest in some of the acoustic nerve fibers innervating mammalian cochlear hair cells (1 to 2 spikes per second).

THE INNER EAR RECEPTOR ORGANS

In the vestibular labyrinth the hair cells are mounted in the macules and cristae, and in the cochlea they are mounted in the organ of Corti. The hair cells function in the same way (as described above) in each of these organs, yet the biologic signals generated are quite different. This difference is due to the mechanical properties of the supporting structures.[18]

The Macule (Fig. 9)

The membranous labyrinth forms two globular cavities within the vestibule, the utricle and saccule (see Figs. 6 and 7). Each cavity contains a separate macule. In the saccule the macule is located on the medial wall in the sagittal plane, while in the utricle the macule is primarily in the horizontal plane next to the opening of the horizontal semicircular canal (Fig. 9C). The surface of the utricular and saccular macules are covered by the otolithic membrane, a structure consisting of a mesh of fibers embedded in a gel with a superficial layer of calcium carbonate crystals, the otoconia (Fig. 9A). The stereocilia of the macular hair cells protrude into the otolithic membrane. The striola, a distinctive curved zone running through the center, divides each macule into two areas. The hair cells on each side of the striola are oriented so that their kinocilia are in opposite directions (as indicated by arrows in Fig. 9C). In the utricle the kinocilia face the striola, and in the saccule they face away from it. Because of this different orientation, displacement of the otolithic membrane has an opposite physiologic influence on the set of hair cells on each side of the striola.

The density of the otolithic membrane overlying the hair cells of the macules is much greater than that of the surrounding endolymph owing to the presence of the calcium carbonate crystals. The weight of this membrane produces a shearing force on the underlying hair cells that is proportional to the sine of the angle between the line of gravitational force and a line perpendicular to the plane of the macule (Fig. 9B). During linear head acceleration tangential

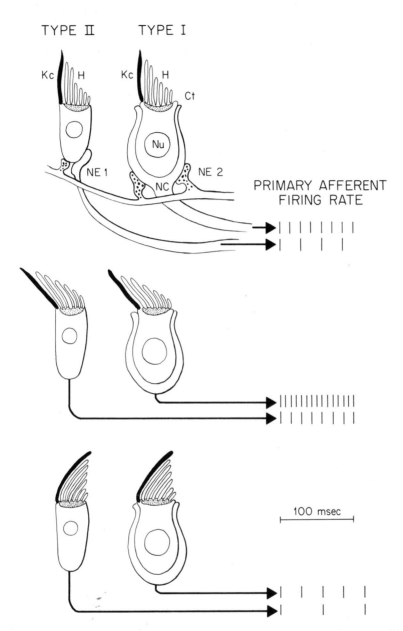

FIGURE 8. Hair cell modulation of spontaneous afferent nerve firing rate. Bending of the stereocilia toward the kinocilium depolarizes the hair cell and increases the firing rate, and bending away from the kinocilium hyperpolarizes the hair cell and decreases the firing rate. Kc—kinocilium, H—hairs, Ct—cuticular plate, Nu—nucleus, NC—nerve chalice, NE—nerve ending (1—afferent, 2—efferent).

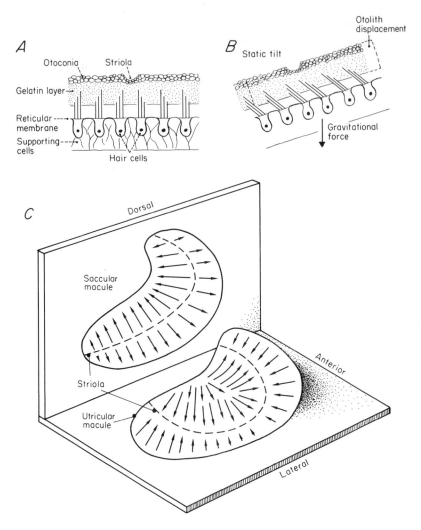

FIGURE 9. The Macule—(A) anatomy, (B) mechanism of hair cell activation with static tilt, and (C) spatial orientation of saccular and utricular macules. Arrows indicate the direction that the kinocilia point toward.

to the surface of the receptor, the force acting on the hair cells is the result of two vector forces: one in the opposite direction of the head displacement, and the other in the direction of gravitational pull. Recordings of afferent neuronal activity from the macules of primates confirm that the utricular and saccular macules are responsive to static tilt and dynamic linear acceleration forces.[19,20,21] The pattern of afferent nerve response is complex, however, with different neurons exhibiting different resting activity, frequency response, and adaptation properties.

The Crista (Fig. 10)

The semicircular canals are aligned to form a coordinate system. The horizontal canal makes a 30-degree angle with a horizontal plane, and the vertical canals make a 45-degree angle with a frontal plane (Fig. 10C).[22] At the anterior opening of the horizontal and anterior semicircular canals and the inferior opening of the posterior semicircular canal, each tube enlarges to form the ampulla (see Fig. 6 and 7). The crista crosses each ampulla in a direction perpendicular to the longitudinal axis of the canal (Fig. 10A). Hair cells are located on the surface of the crista, with their cilia protruding into the cupula, a gelatinous mass of the same composition as the otolithic membrane. The cupula extends from the surface of the crista to the ceiling of the ampulla, forming what appears to be a watertight seal.

The hair cells within each crista are oriented with their kinocilium in the same direction. However, in the horizontal canal the kinocilia are directed toward the utricular side of the ampulla (as in Figs. 10A and B), while in the vertical canals the kinocilia are directed toward the canal side of the ampulla. This difference in morphologic polarization explains the difference in directional sensitivity between the horizontal and vertical canals. The afferent nerve fibers of the horizontal canals increase their baseline firing rate when endolymph moves in the utricular or ampullopetal direction, while those of the vertical canals increase their baseline firing rate with ampullofugal endolymph flow.

Since the cupula has the same specific gravity as the surrounding fluids, it is not subject to displacement by changes in the line of gravitational force. However, the forces associated with angular head acceleration result in a displacement of the cupula and bending of the hair cells of the crista (Fig. 10B). The motion of the cupula can be likened to that of a pendulum in a viscous medium. Sudden displacement of the cupula by a step of angular head acceleration is followed by a gradual exponential return of the cupula to its baseline position. The rate of return is determined by the ratio of the viscous drag coefficient of the endolymph to the elasticity coefficient of the cupula, according to the so-called torsion-pendulum model.[18]

Precise measurements of primary afferent nerve activity originating from the cristae of squirrel monkeys during physiologic rotatory stimulation reveal that the change in frequency of action potentials is approximately proportional to the deviation of the cupula as predicted by the pendulum model.[23,24,25] For example, during sinusoidal head rotation in the plane of a semicircular canal, a sinusoidal change in firing frequency is superimposed on a rather high resting discharge (about 90 spikes per second) (Fig. 11). The peak firing rate occurs at the time of maximum cupular displacement, which occurs at the time of peak angular head velocity. With small amplitude sinusoidal rotation, the modulation is almost symmetrical about the baseline firing rate. For larger stimulus amplitudes the responses become increasingly asymmetrical. The excitatory re-

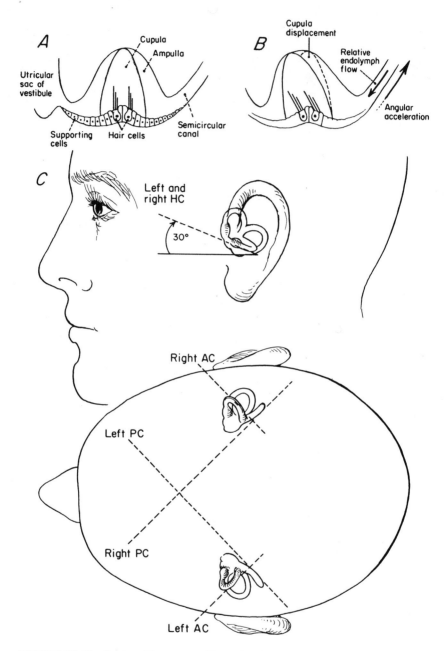

FIGURE 10. The Crista—(A) anatomy, (B) mechanism of hair cell activation with angular acceleration, and (C) orientation of the semicircular canals within the head. HC—horizontal canal, PC—posterior canal, AC—anterior canal.

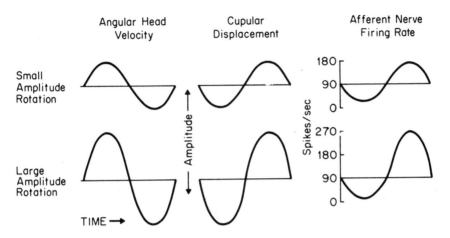

FIGURE 11. Relationship between angular head velocity, cupular displacement, and primary afferent nerve firing rate during sinusoidal angular rotation in the plane of the horizontal semicircular canal. During small amplitude rotation the modulation of afferent nerve activity is approximately symmetrical about the baseline level (approximately 90 spikes per sec), whereas with large amplitude rotation the modulation is markedly asymmetric.

sponses can increase up to 350 to 400 spikes per second in proportion to stimulus magnitude, while the growth of inhibitory response is limited to the disappearance of spontaneous activity. This asymmetry in afferent nerve response partially explains why rotatory induced nystagmus is asymmetric in patients with only one functioning labyrinth (see Rotatory Testing, Chapter 7).[18]

The Organ of Corti (Fig. 12)

The cochlear duct is a spiral membranous canal that subdivides the bony spiral canal of the cochlea into the scala vestibuli and scala tympani (Fig. 12C). The spiral ligament, located in a sulcus on the external wall of the bony cochlear duct, serves as the external attachment of the basilar membrane and Reissner's membrane. The scala media, between Reissner's membrane and the basilar membrane, contains endolymph, while the scala vestibuli and scala tympani contain perilymph (see Fig. 6). The organ of Corti is mounted on the scala media side of the basement membrane.

Hair cells in the organ of Corti contain only stereocilia, being devoid of kinocilia. The stereocilia project into the tectorial membrane, a gelatinous structure overlying the organ of Corti. The ends of the cilia rest within pockets in the tectorial membrane. Upward displacement of the basilar membrane results in a shearing force between the organ of Corti and the tectorial membrane. The hair cells are displaced in relationship to the relatively fixed tectorial membrane (acting as a hinge) (Fig. 12B).

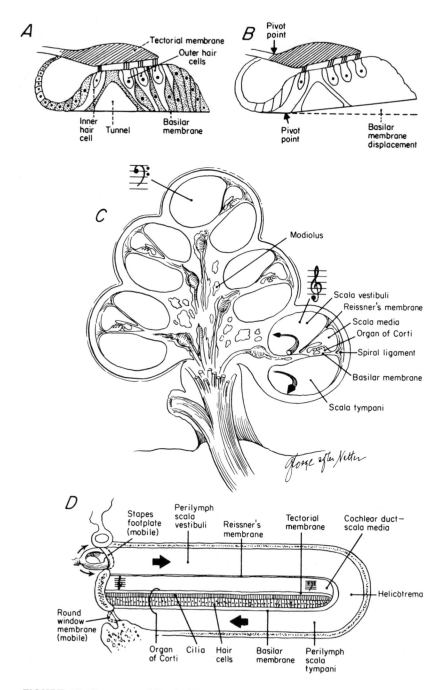

FIGURE 12. The organ of Corti—(A) anatomy, (B) mechanism of hair cell activation with sound-induced basilar membrane displacement, (C) and (D) direction of fluid displacement within the cochlea, in (D) the spiral cochlea has been schematically unwound. Arrows indicate direction of perilymph movement.

Inward movement of the stapes displaces the inner ear fluid toward the round window, resulting in outward movement of the round window membrane (Fig. 12D). This movement of fluid sets into motion a complicated wave form on the basilar membrane, exciting the hair cells of the organ of Corti as described above. According to the traveling wave theory, maximum displacement of the basement membrane occurs at different distances from the stapes depending on the frequency of the sound.[26] For low frequency sounds, maximum displacement occurs near the apex, while for high frequency sound, maximum displacement is closer to the base. Measurements of action potentials from single acoustic nerve fibers reveal a frequency-dependent excitability that resembles the filter properties of the basilar membrane.[27] Each fiber has a characteristic frequency at which it is most sensitive. The sensitivity decays very rapidly for frequencies on either side of this characteristic frequency.

Since frequency has a spatial distribution within the cochlea, lesions involving restricted areas of the cochlea are expressed functionally as threshold losses for different parts of the auditory spectrum. In animals, surgically induced lesions in the apical region cause hearing loss for low frequencies, while lesions of the basal end of the cochlea create severe high frequency hearing losses.[28] Clinical-pathologic studies in patients with hearing loss have documented a similar frequency-spatial distribution within the human cochlea (see Fig. 69).[6]

Unifying Concept of Hair Cell Function

In all cases the effective stimulus to the sensory cells in the labyrinth is the relative displacement of the cilia produced by application of mechanical force to their surroundings. Since the mechanical properties of the "supporting and coupling" structures are different, the frequency ranges at which the cilia can be moved by the applied force also are different. The otolithic membrane is maximally displaced during constant linear acceleration such as that associated with gravity, but its motion rapidly diminishes if the linear acceleration changes at a frequency greater than 0.5 Hz, owing to the characteristics of the restraining visco-elastic forces holding the otolith to the macule. The semicircular canals respond only to angular acceleration at frequencies below 5 Hz, owing to the inertial and viscous forces restraining the displacement of fluid and cupula in the narrow semicircular canals. Because of the great flexibility of the basilar membrane, the range of sound frequencies to which the hair cells in the cochlea are sensitive varies from 20 to 20,000 Hz.

THE EIGHTH NERVE

The eighth nerve, a combination of the auditory and vestibular nerves, enters the posterior cranial fossa through the internal auditory canal (Fig. 13). The auditory nerve, consisting of approximately 30,000 fibers, occupies the anterior-inferior part of the internal auditory canal, and the vestibular nerve, containing approximately 20,000 fibers, occupies the posterior half. The facial nerve is located in the remaining anterior superior quadrant.

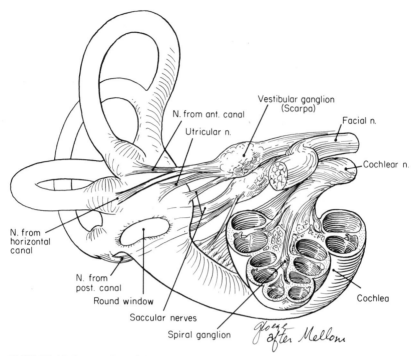

FIGURE 13. Innervation of the labyrinth.

The afferent bipolar ganglion cells of the vestibular nerve (Scarpa's ganglion) are arranged in two cell masses in a vertical column within the internal auditory canal, the superior group forming the superior division of the vestibular nerve, and the inferior group forming the inferior division. The superior division innervates the cristae of the anterior and horizontal canals, the macule of the utricle, and the anterior superior part of the macule of the saccule. The inferior division innervates the crista of the posterior canal and the main portion of the saccule. The bipolar cochlear neurons are located in the spiral ganglion of the cochlea. As with the vestibular nerve, the orderly spatial arrangement of the cochlear neurons within the spiral ganglion is maintained in the nerve trunk. The nerve fibers from the basal turn of the cochlea are located in the peripheral and inferior portions of the nerve trunk, and the apical fibers are in the central region.

REFERENCES

1. GRAY, O: *A brief survey of the phylogenesis of the labyrinth.* J Laryngol Otol 69:151, 1955.
2. WERSALL, DJ, AND BAGGER-SJOBACK, D: *Morphology of the vestibular sense*

organs. In KORNHUBER, HH (ED): *Handbook fo Sensory Physiology, vol VI, part 2.* Springer-Verlag, New York, 1974.

3. BAIRD, LL: *Some aspects of the comparative anatomy and evolution of the inner ear in submammalian vertebrates.* In RISS, W (ED): *Brain, Behavior and Evolution.* S Karger, Basel, 1974.

4. PEARSON, AA: *The Development of the Ear: A Manual.* Rochester, MN. American Academy of Ophthalmology and Otolaryngology, 1967.

5. DOHLMAN, GF: *The mechanism of secretion and absorption of endolymph in the vestibular apparatus.* Acta Otolaryngol (Stockh) 59:275, 1965.

6. SCHUKNECHT, HF: *Pathology of the Ear.* Harvard University Press, Cambridge, MA, 1974.

7. KIMURA, R, SCHUKNECHT, H, AND OTA, C: *Blockage of the cochlear aqueduct.* Acta Otolaryngol (Stockh) 77:1, 1974.

8. LUNDQUIST, PG: *The endolymphatic duct and sac in the guinea pig.* Acta Otolaryngol 201 (Suppl) (Stockh):1, 1965.

9. KIMURA, RS: *Experimental production of endolymphatic hydrops.* In PULEC, J (ED): *Meniere's Disease.* WB Saunders, Philadelphia, 1968.

10. SUH, KW, AND CODY, DTR: *Obliteration of vestibular and cochlear aqueducts in animals.* Trans Amer Acad Ophthalmol Otolaryngol 84:359, 1977.

11. PAPARELLA, M: *Biochemical Mechanisms in Hearing and Deafness.* Charles C Thomas, Springfield, IL, 1970.

12. SCHUKNECHT, H, AND EL SEIFI, A: *Experimental observations on the fluid physiology of the inner ear.* Ann Otol Rhinol Laryngol 72:687, 1963.

13. MAZZONI, A: *Internal auditory artery supply to the petrous bone.* Ann Otol Rhinol Laryngol 81:13, 1974.

14. PERLMAN, HB, KIMURA, RS, AND FERNANDEZ, C: *Experiments on temporary obstruction of the internal auditory artery.* Laryngoscope 69:591, 1959.

15. FLOCK, A: *Sensory transduction in hair cells.* In LOWENSTEIN, WR (ED): *Handbook of Sensory Physiology, Principles of Receptor Physiology, vol 1.* Springer-Verlag, New York, 1971.

16. SHOTWELL, SL, JOCOBS, R, HUDSPETH, AJ: *Directional sensitivity of individual vertebrate hair cells to controlled deflection of their hair bundles.* In COHEN, B (ED): *Vestibular and Oculomotor Physiology.* Ann NY Acad Sciences 374:1, 1981.

17. LOWENSTEIN, OE: *Comparative morphology and physiology.* In KORNHUBER, HH (ED): *Handbook of Sensory Physiology, vol VI, part 2.* Springer-Verlag, New York, 1974.

18. BALOH, RW, HONRUBIA, V: *Clinical Neurophysiology of the Vestibular System.* FA Davis, Philadelphia, 1979.

19. FERNANDEZ, C, AND GOLDBERG, JM: *Physiology of peripheral neurons innervating otolith organs of the squirrel monkey. I. Response to static tilts and to long-duration centrifugal force.* J Neurophysiol 39:970, 1976.

20. FERNANDEZ, C, AND GOLDBERG, JM: *Physiology of peripheral neurons innervating otolith organs of the squirrel monkey. II. Directional selectivity and force-response relations.* J Neurophysiol 39:985, 1976.

21. FERNANDEZ, C, AND GOLDBERG, JM: *Physiology of peripheral neurons innervating otolith organs of the squirrel monkey. III. Response dynamics.* J Neurophysiol 39:996, 1976.

22. BLANKS, RHI, CURTHOYS, IS, AND MARKHAM, CH: *Planar relationships of the semicircular canals in man.* Acta Otolaryngol (Stockh) 80:185, 1975.

23. GOLDBERG, J, AND FERNANDEZ, C: *Physiology of peripheral neurons innervating semicircular canals of the squirrel monkey. I. Resting discharge and response to constant angular accelerations.* J Neurophysiol 34:635, 1971.

24. FERNANDEZ, C, AND GOLDBERG, JM: *Physiology of peripheral neurons innervating semicircular canals of the squirrel monkey. II. Response to sinusoidal stimulation and dynamics of peripheral system.* J Neurophysiol 34:661, 1971.

25. GOLDBERG, JM, AND FERNANDEZ, C: *Physiology of peripheral neurons innervating semicircular canals of the squirrel monkey. III. Variations among units in their discharge properties.* J Neurophysiol 34:676, 1971.

26. BEKESY, G VON: *Experiments in Hearing.* McGraw-Hill, New York, 1960.

27. TASAKI, I: *Afferent impulses in auditory nerve fibers and the mechanism of impulse initiation in the cochlea.* In RASMUSSEN, G, AND WINDLE, W (EDS): *Neural Mechanisms of the Auditory and Vestibular System.* Charles C Thomas, Springfield, IL, 1960.

28. SUTTON, S, AND SCHUKNECHT, H: *Regional hearing loss from induced cochlear injuries in experimental animals.* Ann Otol Rhinol Laryngol 63:727, 1954.

3

THE CENTRAL
VESTIBULAR SYSTEM

THE VESTIBULAR NUCLEI

VESTIBULO-OCULAR REFLEXES
General Organization
Canal-Ocular Connections
Nystagmus
Otolith-Ocular Connections
Interaction with Visual and Neck Proprioceptive Signals

VESTIBULOSPINAL REFLEXES
Lateral Vestibulospinal Tract
Medial Vestibulospinal Tract
Reticulospinal Tract
Cerebellar-Vestibular Pathways
Vestibular Influence on Posture and Equilibrium

VESTIBULOCORTICAL PROJECTIONS

THE VESTIBULAR EFFERENT SYSTEM

THE VESTIBULAR NUCLEI

The central processes of the primary afferent vestibular neurons divide into an ascending and descending branch after entering the brainstem at the inner aspect of the restiform body (Fig. 14).[1] The ascending branch ends either in the rostral end of the vestibular nuclei or in the cerebellum, while the descending branch ends in the caudal vestibular nuclei. The vestibular nuclei consist of a

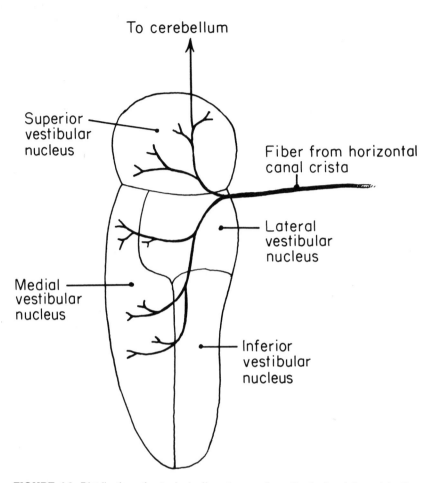

FIGURE 14. Distribution of a typical afferent nerve from the horizontal semicircular canal within the vestibular nuclei. (Adapted from Gacek, R: *The course and central termination of first order neurons supplying vestibular end organs in the cat.* Acta Otolaryngol Suppl 254, 1969).

group of neurons located on the floor of the fourth ventricle bounded laterally by the restiform body, ventrally by the nucleus and spinal tract of the trigeminal nerve, and medially by the pontine reticular formation.[2] Four distinct anatomic groups of neurons have traditionally been identified: the medial, lateral, superior, and inferior nuclei (see Fig. 14). Although there is considerable overlap, the majority of fibers originating from the utricle and saccule end in the lateral and inferior nuclei, while most fibers originating from the semicircular canals terminate in the superior and medial nuclei. In addition to the vestibular afferent projections, the vestibular nuclei receive signals from the cerebellum, the cervical spinal cord, and the nearby reticular formation. There are also large numbers of interconnecting commissural fibers between the vestibular nuclei on both sides. Based on the combined afferent and efferent fiber connections, the lateral and inferior vestibular nuclei are important relay stations for the control of vestibulospinal reflexes, while the superior and medial nuclei are critical stations for control of the vestibulo-ocular reflexes.

VESTIBULO-OCULAR REFLEXES

General Organization

Connections between the vestibular nuclei and the oculomotor neurons run in two separate pathways: one is a direct pathway from secondary vestibular neurons to oculomotor neurons, and the other is an indirect pathway relayed through the reticular substance of the brainstem.[3,4] Many of the direct connections from the vestibular nuclei to the oculomotor nuclei are part of a large fiber bundle, the medial longitudinal fasciculus (MLF), lying along the floor of the fourth ventricle. This fiber bundle extends from the cervical cord to the reticular substance of the midbrain and thalamus, providing an interconnecting pathway between the vestibular and the abducens nuclei in the middle brainstem, and the oculomotor complex in the rostral brainstem. The indirect pathway between the vestibular and oculomotor nuclei is multisynaptic, involving both short and long axonal interconnections within the reticular substance.

Precise vestibulo-ocular control requires the combination of activity in both pathways. Vestibulo-ocular reflexes are reduced, but not abolished, by sectioning the axons in the MLF, or by lesions in the pontine reticular formation.[5,6] The MFL and reticular pathways complement each other, the former providing a quick communication channel and the latter acting as a modulator. By way of reverberating circuits, the reticular formation maintains a level of spontaneous activity, or tonus, and integrates information from several neural centers. It creates the necessary delays for summation of signals from the visual, proprioceptive, and vestibular systems to produce accurate compensatory eye movements. It acts, therefore, as a fine tuner of vestibular-induced eye movements.

Canal-Ocular Connections

The afferent nerves from each semicircular canal are connected to the motor neurons of the eye muscles in such a way that stimulation of the nerve from a given canal results in eye movement in the plane of that canal.[7] For example, stimulation of the ampullary nerve from the left posterior canal causes excitation of the ipsilateral superior oblique and contralateral inferior rectus muscles, while inhibiting the ipsilateral inferior oblique and the contralateral superior rectus. An oblique downward movement in the plane of the left posterior canal is the end result.

The direct pathways from the horizontal canals to the horizontal extraocular muscles (Fig. 15) deserve particular attention, since the horizontal vestibulo-

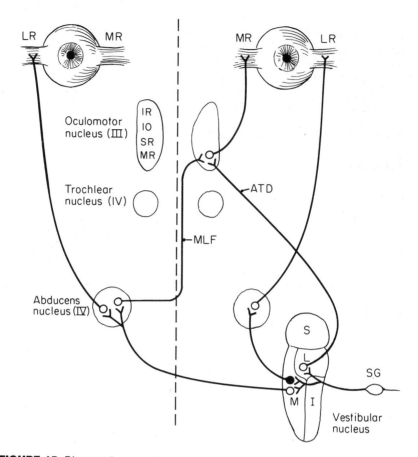

FIGURE 15. Direct pathways of the horizontal semicircular canal-ocular reflex. Darkened cell body indicates an inhibitory secondary vestibular neuron; SG—Scarpa's ganglion, S—superior nucleus, L—lateral nucleus, M—medial nucleus, I—inferior nucleus, MLF—medial longitudinal fasciculus, ATD—ascending tract of Dieters, IR—inferior rectus, IO—inferior oblique, SR—superior rectus, MR—medial rectus, LR—lateral rectus.

ocular reflex is the focus of many clinical vestibular tests. The secondary vestibular neurons lie in the medial and lateral vestibular nucleus.[1,8] The more medial group of excitatory neurons project to the contralateral abducens nucleus, while the more laterally located excitatory neurons (in the medial part of the lateral nucleus) project to ipsilateral medial rectus motoneurons via the ascending tract of Deiters (ATD). The ipsilateral medial rectus neurons also receive a strong excitatory input via the medial longitudinal fasciculus (MLF) from interneurons in the contralateral abducens nucleus. These interneurons are excited by the same secondary vestibular neurons that excite the abducens motor neurons.[9] The relative contribution to the horizontal vestibulo-ocular reflex of the ATD and

MLF excitatory pathways is not entirely clear. However, the MLF pathway seems most important, since the eyes cannot adduct past the midline if the MLF is sectioned.[6] Inhibitory secondary neurons in the rostral part of the medial vestibular nucleus run directly to the ipsilateral abducens nucleus. Contralateral medial rectus motoneurons apparently do not receive disynaptic inhibition from the horizontal semicircular canals.[8,9]

In addition to the direct and indirect connections between secondary vestibular neurons and oculomotor neurons, commissural connections between the two vestibular nuclei play an important role in controlling the vestibulo-ocular reflex.[10] Through inhibitory interneurons, secondary vestibular neurons on one side inhibit their counterpart on the opposite side. The commissural connections are particularly important after unilateral loss of vestibular function, since they provide a mechanism for a single labyrinth to control the vestibular nuclei on both sides, thus maintaining a functional vestibulo-ocular reflex (see Exercises and Vestibular Compensation, Chapter 12).

Because physiologic stimuli activate both labyrinths, the horizontal vestibulo-ocular reflex is controlled by a four-way, push-pull mechanism.[4] For example, physiologic stimulation of the crista of the right horizontal semicircular canal excites the left lateral rectus and the right medial rectus and inhibits the right lateral rectus. Because of the symmetry between the labyrinths, the same receptor in the other ear simultaneously diminishes its afferent output, thereby disfacilitating the left medial rectus and right lateral rectus, and disinhibiting the left lateral rectus. The end result is contraction of the left lateral and right medial rectus muscles and relaxation of the left medial and right lateral rectus muscles.

Nystagmus

If a subject is rotated back and forth in the dark in the plane of the horizontal semicircular canals, compensatory eye movements are induced with eye velocity approximately equal and opposite to the head velocity.[4] If the angle of rotation is large, such that it cannot be compensated for by motion of the eye in the orbit, the slow compensatory vestibular-induced eye deviation is interrupted by quick movements in the opposite direction. This combination of rhythmic slow and fast eye movements is called nystagmus. Because of the fast components, the trajectory of the eye motion during the slow components effectively compensates for head rotation as if the eye had unlimited freedom of motion. Without the fast components the eyes would become pinned in an extreme orbital position and the vestibulo-ocular reflex would cease functioning.

Spontaneous nystagmus occurs after lesions of the labyrinth, the vestibular nerve and the central vestibulo-ocular neurons, and interconnecting pathways.[4] The key ingredient for the production of spontaneous nystagmus is an imbalance of tonic signals within the vestibulo-ocular pathways. Damage to one labyrinth or one vestibular nerve results in spontaneous nystagmus, with the slow phase directed toward the side of the lesion; the tonic input from the intact side is no longer balanced by input from the damaged side. This spontaneous nystagmus is indistinguishable from nystagmus produced by physiologic stimulation of the opposite normal vestibular nerve (Fig. 16). The direction of spontaneous nystagmus associated with lesions in the brainstem is less predictable, depending on the location and extent of the lesion.[11] Central spontaneous nystagmus can be purely vertical or torsional, since tonic signals to the oblique and vertical rectus muscles run in separate pathways from the vestibular nuclei.[12]

Groups of neurons in the paramedian pontine reticular formation (PPRF) immediately adjacent to the abducens nuclei fire in short bursts of activity just before the onset of horizontal fast components.[13,14] Numerous pathways interconnect neurons in the vestibular nuclei with neurons in this region of the PPRF, and the latter project directly to oculomotor neurons and interneurons in the abducens nucleus. Apparently neurons in the PPRF monitor vestibulo-ocular signals and intermittently fire in bursts to produce corrective fast components based on certain features of the signal, particularly the eye position in the orbit. During angular rotation the fast components of the initial beats of nystagmus attain a larger amplitude than the preceding slow components, and the eyes deviate in the direction of the fast component.[4] The apparent advantage of this strategy is that the eyes are ready to focus on newly arriving targets in the field of rotation, and fixation can be maintained during the subsequent slow component. Unilateral lesions of the PPRF impair ipsilateral rapid eye movements, and the eyes deviate to the contralateral side of the orbit.[15] Stimuli that normally would produce nystagmus with ipsilateral fast components simply cause a strong tonic contralateral deviation of the eyes.

Otolith-Ocular Connections

The pathways from the macules to the extraocular muscles are less clearly defined than those from the semicircular canals.[1,8] Because of the varied orientation of hair cells within the macules (see Fig. 9), simultaneous stimulation of all the nerve fibers coming from a macule produces a nonphysiologic excitation, and the induced eye movements fail to represent the naturally occurring ones.[7] Selective stimulation of different parts of the utricle and saccule results in mostly vertical and vertical-rotatory eye movements. As one would expect, stimulation on each side of the striola produces oppositely directed rotatory and vertical components.

Each of the vertical eye muscles appears to be connected to specific areas of the macules, so that groups of hair cells whose kinocilia are oriented in opposite directions excite agonist and antagonist muscles. Lateral tilt of the head produces countertorsional eye movements, while forward-backward tilt results in vertical rotation (Fig. 17). Otolith-ocular reflexes in normal human subjects are inefficient and variable.[16,17] For example, the maximum ocular torsion for lateral tilt of 50 degrees is only about 5 or 6 degrees (i.e., a gain of approximately 0.1).

Interaction with Visual and Neck Proprioceptive Signals

Visual, proprioceptive, and vestibular signals interact synergistically to stabilize gaze during most natural head movements.[4] The effect is better ocular stability

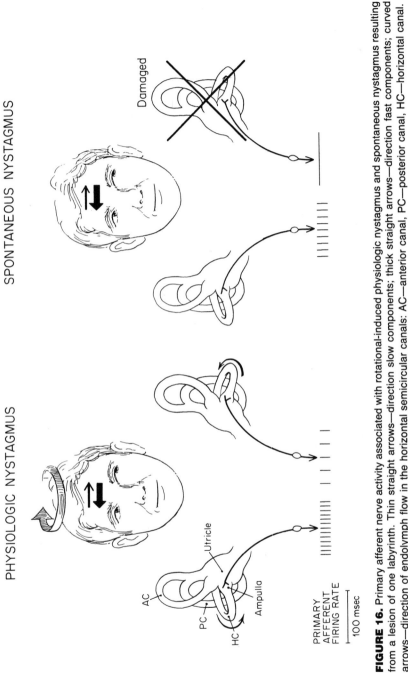

FIGURE 16. Primary afferent nerve activity associated with rotational-induced physiologic nystagmus and spontaneous nystagmus resulting from a lesion of one labyrinth. Thin straight arrows—direction slow components; thick straight arrows—direction fast components; curved arrows—direction of endolymph flow in the horizontal semicircular canals: AC—anterior canal, PC—posterior canal, HC—horizontal canal.

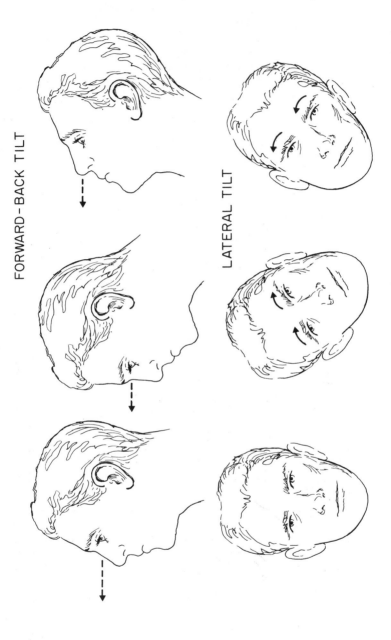

FORWARD – BACK TILT

LATERAL TILT

FIGURE 17. Otolith-ocular reflexes induced by forward-backward tilt and lateral tilt.

than would be possible if each system worked alone. Occasionally these signals conflict, and one must override the others in order to maintain gaze stability. For example, when the head and visual target are moving at the same velocity, the vestibulo-ocular and nuchal ocular reflexes are suppressed and gaze is maintained on the target.

Secondary vestibular neurons receive afferent visual and proprioceptive signals in addition to primary vestibular signals (Fig. 18). The visual and proprioceptive signals are organized such that movement of the visual surround in one direction excites and inhibits the same neurons that are excited and inhibited by movement of the head and neck in the opposite direction. The vestibular nucleus is therefore not simply a relay station for vestibular reflexes, but rather an important sensorimotor interaction center.

Visual signals reach the vestibular nuclei by at least two different pathways: a cortical pathway with relay stations in the geniculate ganglion and parieto-occipital cortex, and a subcortical pathway with relay stations in the pretectum.[18,19] Details on the exact pathways to the vestibular nuclei from these visual centers are poorly understood, but the cerebellum (particularly the flocculonodular lobes) appears to be a critical relay station for both pathways. Monkeys who have undergone flocculectomy and humans with midline cerebellar lesions are unable to inhibit vestibular signals with visual signals.[20,21] Floccular Purkinje cells receive primary vestibular afferent signals and visual signals, and in turn send out impulses to second-order neurons of the vestibulo-ocular reflex arc.[22] Apparently the flocculus "compares" visual and vestibular signals, and if the signals are in conflict with each other, the characteristics of the vestibular response is changed at the level of the vestibular nucleus.

Neck proprioceptive signals originate from receptors deep in the ligaments and joints of the upper cervical vertebrae (C1–C3) and interact at the vestibular nucleus with afferent vestibular signals (see Fig. 18).[4,23] Stimulation of the neck joint receptors activates neurons in the contralateral vestibular nucleus that are part of the canal-ocular pathways. Turning the head to the right stretches the joint ligaments and thereby activates receptors in the left side of the neck. This activity excites neurons in the right vestibular nucleus, which in turn excites neurons in the left abducens nucleus and right oculomotor nucleus. Inhibitory interneurons in the vestibular nuclei are also activated by afferent nerve signals from the neck to maintain the necessary balance between excitation of agonist muscles and inhibition of antagonist muscles. Unilateral interruption of cervical proprioceptive signals by either root section or local anesthetic block produces nystagmus in animals and vertigo in human subjects.[24] However, compared with the labyrinthine input to the vestibular nuclei, cervical input is minor, and its interruption results in relatively mild functional loss that is rapidly compensated for (see Cervical Vertigo, Chapter 9).

VESTIBULOSPINAL REFLEXES

Secondary vestibular neurons influence spinal anterior horn cell activity by means of three major pathways: (1) the lateral vestibulospinal tract, (2) the me-

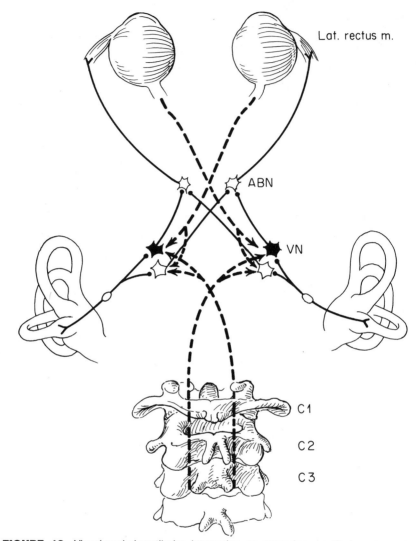

FIGURE 18. Visual-nuchal-vestibular interaction at secondary vestibular neurons within the horizontal semicircular canal ocular reflex. ABN—abducens neurons, VN—vestibular nucleus neurons; black—inhibitory neuron, white—excitatory neuron.

dial vestibulospinal tract, and (3) the reticulospinal tract.[1,25] The first two arise directly from neurons in the vestibular nuclei (Fig. 19), while the third arises from neurons in the reticular formation that are influenced by vestibular stimulation (as well as several other kinds of input). The cerebellum is highly interrelated with each of these pathways.

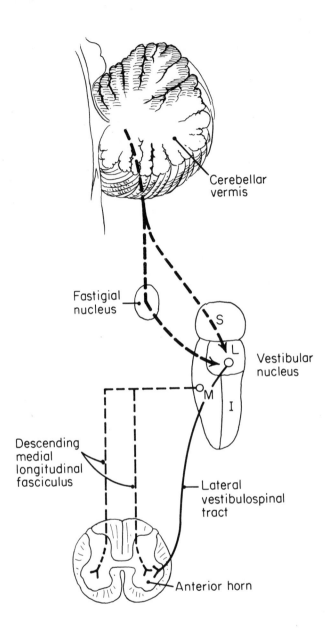

FIGURE 19. Vestibulospinal pathways: Thin dashed lines represent multisynaptic connections of the medial vestibulospinal tract, heavy dashed lines represent the strong influence of the cerebellar vermis on secondary vestibular neurons, giving rise to the lateral vestibulospinal tract.

Lateral Vestibulospinal Tract

The majority of fibers in the lateral vestibulospinal tract originate from neurons in the lateral vestibular nucleus.[25] A somatotopic pattern of projections originates in the lateral vestibular nucleus such that neurons in the rostroventral region supply the cervical cord, while neurons in the dorsocaudal region innervate the lumbosacral cord. Neurons in the intermediate region supply the thoracic cord. Although the lateral vestibulospinal tract is largely uncrossed, a small component of the pathway reaches the contralateral gray matter via the spinal ventral gray commissure. Electric stimulation in the lateral nucleus produces monosynaptic excitation of ipsilateral extensor motoneurons and disynaptic inhibition of contralateral flexor motoneurons.

Medial Vestibulospinal Tract

The fibers of the medial vestibulospinal tract originate from neurons in the medial vestibular nucleus and enter the spinal cord in the descending MLF.[25] The fibers travel in the ventral funicle as far as the midthoracic level. The majority end on interneurons in the cervical cord. No monosynaptic connections appear to exist between the medial vestibulospinal tract and cervical anterior horn cells.

Reticulospinal Tract

The reticulospinal tract originates from neurons in the bulbar reticular formation.[25] The nuclei reticularis gigantocellularis and pontis caudalis provide most of the long fibers passing into the spinal cord, although the majority of neurons in the caudal reticular formation also contribute fibers. Only a small number of primary vestibular fibers end in the reticular formation, so that the main vestibular influence on reticulospinal outflow is mediated by way of the secondary vestibular neurons. A pattern exists within the vestibuloreticular projections such that each nucleus projects to different areas of the reticular formation, but no detailed somatotopic organization has been identified. Both crossed and uncrossed fibers traverse the length of the spinal cord. Stimulation of the pontomedullary reticular formation in the regions where the long descending spinal projections originate results in inhibition of both extensor and flexor motoneurons throughout the spinal cord.

Cerebellar-Vestibular Pathways

The midline or "spinal" cerebellum provides a major source of input to neurons whose axons form the lateral vestibulospinal and reticulospinal tracts.[26] A somatotopic organization of projections to the lateral nucleus occurs in both the vermian cortex and fastigial nuclei. Direct projections connect the vermian cortex to the lateral vestibular nucleus, and indirect projections pass through the fastigial nuclei (see Fig. 19). The caudal part of the fastigial nucleus gives rise to a bundle of fibers that crosses the midline (Russell's hook bundle), curving around the brachium conjunctivum before running to the contralateral lateral vestibular nucleus and dorsolateral reticular formation. In addition, direct ipsilateral outflow passes from the fastigial nucleus to areas of the reticular formation that send long fibers to the spinal cord in the reticulospinal tract. The cerebellar-reticular pathways do not exhibit somatotopic organization.

The cerebellar vermis and fastigial nuclei receive input from secondary vestibular neurons, the spinal cord, and the pontomedullary reticular formation. The result is a close knit vestibular-reticular-cerebellar functional unit for the maintenance of equilibrium and locomotion.[27]

Vestibular Influence on Posture and Equilibrium

The anterior horn cells of the antigravity muscles (extensors of the neck, trunk and extremities) are under the combined excitatory and inhibitory influence of multiple supraspinal neural centers.[4] At least in the cat, one finds two main facilitatory centers (the lateral vestibular nucleus and rostral reticular formation), and four inhibitory centers (the pericruciate cortex, basal ganglia, cerebellum, and caudal reticular formation). The balance of input from these different centers determines the degree of tone in the antigravity muscles. If one removes the inhibitory influence of the frontal cortex and basal ganglia by sectioning the animal's midbrain, a characteristic state of contraction in the antigravity muscles results, so-called decerebrate rigidity. The extensor muscles increase their resistance to lengthening, and the deep tendon reflexes become hyperactive. The vestibular system contributes largely to this increased extensor tone, since it markedly decreases after bilateral destruction of the labyrinths. Unilateral destruction of the labyrinth or the lateral vestibular nucleus results in an ipsilateral decrease in tone, indicating that the main excitatory input to the anterior horn cells arrives from the ipsilateral lateral vestibulospinal tract.

In a decerebrate animal with normal labyrinths, the intensity of the extensor tone can be modulated in a specific way by changing the position of the head in space. The tone is maximal when the animal is in the supine position with the angle of the mouth 45 degrees above horizontal, and minimal when the animal is prone with the angle of the mouth 45 degrees below the horizontal. Intermediate positions of rotation of the animal's body about the transverse or longitudinal axis result in intermediate degrees of extensor tone. If the head of the upright animal is tilted upward, extensor tone in the forelegs increases; downward tilting of the head causes decreased extensor tone and flexion of the forelegs. Lateral tilt produces extension of the extremities on the opposite side.

These tonic labyrinthine reflexes, mediated by way of the otoliths, seldom occur in intact animals or human subjects because of the inhibitory influence of the higher cortical and subcortical centers. They can be demonstrated in premature infants, however, and in adults with lesions releasing the brainstem from the higher neural centers.[28]

VESTIBULOCORTICAL PROJECTIONS

Several clinical observations support the existence of a specific vestibular sensation.[4] Patients without vestibular function (on either an acquired or congenital basis) do not experience a turning sensation when rotated in the dark if visual and tactile cues are eliminated. Patients with complete spinal transections in the cervical region, on the other hand, perceive acceleration of the head and body normally. The sensation of movement is not dependent on vision or associated nystagmus, since blind subjects and patients with complete oculomotor paralysis experience a spinning sensation comparable to that of normal subjects when their vestibular end organs are stimulated. Epileptic discharges from many different areas of the cortex can be associated with a subjective illusion of movement (usually spinning), implying a cerebrocortical representation for vestibular sensation.

The ascending vestibulocortical system includes at least three synaptic stations: the vestibular nuclei, the thalamus, and the cerebral cortex.[8] Vestibulothalamic projections originate from neurons in the superior and lateral vestibular nuclei. At least two thalamic regions receive projections from these secondary vestibular neurons.[8,29] A large anterior vestibulothalamic projection runs ventrally in the brainstem, passing lateral to the red nucleus and dorsal to the subthalamic nucleus, to terminate in the main sensory nucleus of the thalamus (nucleus ventralis posterior lateralis pars oralis) (Fig. 20). A smaller posterior vestibulothalamic projection runs in the lateral lemniscus along with the auditory projections, and ends predominantly near the medial geniculate. The vast majority of vestibulothalamic projections run outside the MLF. Two separate thalamocortical projection areas have been identified in the monkey: one near the central sulcus close to the motor cortex, and the other at the lower end of the intraparietal sulcus next to the face area of the post central gyrus.[30] In humans, electrical stimulation of the superior sylvian gyrus and the region of the inferior intraparietal sulcus produces a subjective sensation of rotation or body displacement.[31]

The vestibulocortical pathway via the thalamus is concerned with the control of body position and orientation in space. Thalamic and cortical units that receive vestibular signals are also activated by proprioception and visual stimuli (as shown in Fig. 20). Most units respond in a similar way to rotation in the dark, or to moving visual fields, indicating that they play a role in relaying information about self motion. From a functional point of view the vestibulothalamocortical projections appear to integrate vestibular, proprioceptive, and visual signals to provide one with a "conscious awareness" of body orientation. Beginning at the vestibular nuclei, a stepwise integration of body orienting signals occurs, reaching its maximum at the level of the cortex.

THE VESTIBULAR EFFERENT SYSTEM

Peripheral vestibular efferent fibers originate from approximately 300 neurons located bilaterally ventromedial to the ventral portion of the lateral vestibular

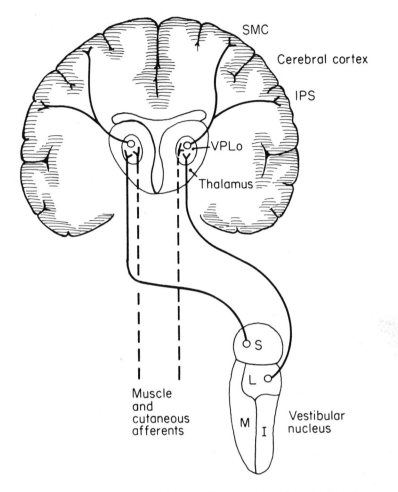

FIGURE 20. Vestibulothalamocortical projections. S—superior nucleus, L—lateral nucleus, M—medial nucleus, I—inferior nucleus, VPLo—nucleus ventralis posterior lateralis pars oralis, IPS—intraparietal sulcus, SMC—sensorimotor cortex.

nucleus.[32] These fibers accompany the cochlear efferent fibers (the so-called olivocochlear bundle) in the vestibular nerve trunk as far as the saccular ganglion, at which point the two efferent systems diverge almost at right angles to each other. Vestibular efferent fibers join each division of the vestibular nerve and run to each macule and crista. Here they end as vesiculated boutons containing many small homogenous vesicles (see Fig. 8). One efferent fiber gives off numerous boutons that will synapse either directly on hair cells or onto their afferent nerve endings. Pharmacologically the efferent fibers and their terminals contain a high concentration of the enzyme acetylcholinesterase, indicating that acetylcholine is probably the peripheral synaptic transmitter.

The functional significance of the vestibular efferent system in man is yet to be determined. Studies in the cat and frog suggest a tonic inhibitory influence of the efferent system on spontaneous afferent activity.[33] However, in the monkey electrical excitation of the central efferent pathways (ipsilateral or contralateral) increases the afferent background activity monitored in Scarpa's ganglion.[34] Thus, there may be species differences in the role of the vestibular efferent system, or the system may have a dual influence upon the hair cells of the vestibular epithelium: one inhibitory and the other excitatory.[35]

REFERENCES

1. GACEK, RR: *The anatomical-physiological basis of vestibular function.* In HONRUBIA, V, AND BRAZIER, MA (EDS): *Nystagmus and Vertigo.* Academic Press, New York, 1982.

2. BRODAL, A: *Anatomy of the vestibular nuclei and their connections.* In KORNHUBER, HH (ED): *Handbook of Sensory Physiology, vol VI, part I.* Springer-Verlag, New York, 1974.

3. LORENTE DE NO, R: *Vestibulo-ocular reflex arc.* Arch Neurol Psychiat 30:245, 1933.

4. BALOH, RW, AND HONRUBIA, V: *Clinical Neurophysiology of the Vestibular System.* FA Davis, Philadelphia, 1979.

5. LORENTE DE NO, R: *The regulation of eye positions and movements induced by the labyrinth.* Laryngoscope 42:233, 1932.

6. EVINGER, LC, FUCHS, AF, AND BAKER, R: *Bilateral lesions of the medial longitudinal fasciculus in monkeys: Effects on the horizontal and vertical components of voluntary and vestibular induced eye movements.* Exp Brain Res 28:1, 1977.

7. COHEN, B: *The vestibulo-ocular reflex arc.* In KORNHUBER, HH (ED): *Handbook of Sensory physiology. The Vestibular System, vol. VI, part 1.* Springer-Verlag, New York, 1974.

8. BUTTNER-ENNEVER, JA: *Vestibular oculomotor organization.* In FUCHS, AF, AND BECKER, W (EDS): *The Neural Control of Eye Movements.* Elsevier, Amsterdam, 1981.

9. BAKER, R, AND HIGHSTEIN, SM: *Vestibular projections to medial rectus subdivision of oculomotor nucleus.* J Neurophysiol 41:1629, 1978.

10. PRECHT, W: *The physiology of the vestibular nuclei.* In KORNHUBER, HH (ED) *Handbook of Sensory Physiology. The Vestibular System, vol. VI, part 1.* Springer-Verlag, New York, 1974.

11. UEMURA, T, AND COHEN, B: *Effects of vestibular nuclei lesions on vestibulo-ocular reflexes and posture in monkeys.* Acta Otolaryngol Suppl 315 (Stockh), 1973.

12. BALOH, RW, AND SPOONER, J: *Downbeat nystagmus: A type of central vestibular nystagmus.* Neurology 31:304, 1981.

13. HENN, V, AND COHEN, B: *Activity in eye motoneurons and brain stem units during eye movements.* In LENNERSTRAND, G, AND BACH-Y-RITA, P (EDS): *Basic Mechanisms of Ocular Motility and their Clinical Implications.* Pergamon Press, Stockholm, 1975.

14. KELLER, EL: *Participation of medial pontine reticular formation in eye movement generation in monkey.* J Neurophysiol 37:316, 1974.

15. HENN, V, AND BUTTNER, V: *Disorders of horizontal gaze.* In LENNERSTRAND, G, ZEE, DS, AND KELLER, EL (EDS): *Functional Basis of Ocular Motility Disorders.* Pergamon Press, New York, 1982.

16. MILLER, EF 2ND: *Counterrolling of the human eye produced by head tilt with respect to gravity.* Acta Otolaryngol (Stockh) 54:479, 1962.

17. DIAMOND, SG, AND MARKHAM, CH: *Binocular counterrolling in humans with unilateral labyrinthectomy and in normal controls.* In *Vestibular and Oculomotor Physiology.* Ann NY Acad Sciences 374:69, 1981.

18. HOFFMANN, KP: *Cortical versus subcortical contributions to the optokinetic reflex in cat.* In LENNERSTRAND, G, ZEE, DS, AND KELLER, EL (EDS): *Functional Basis of Ocular Motility Disorders.* Pergamon Press, New York, 1982.

19. BALOH, RW, YEE, RD, AND HONRUBIA, V: *Clinical abnormalities of optokinetic nystagmus.* In LENNERSTRAND, G, ZEE, D, AND KELLER, EL (EDS): *Functional Basis of Ocular Motility Disorders.* Pergamon Press, Oxford and New York, 1982.

20. ZEE, DS: *Ocular motor abnormalities related to lesions in the vestibulocerebellum in primate.* In LENNERSTRAND, G, ZEE, D, AND KELLER, EL (EDS): *Functional Basis of Ocular Motility Disorders.* Pergamon Press, Oxford and New York, 1982.

21. BALOH, RW, YEE, RD, KIMM, J, AND HONRUBIA, V: *The vestibulo-ocular reflex in patients with lesions involving the vestibulocerebellum.* Exp Neurol 72:141, 1981.

22. MILES, FA, AND FULLER, JH: *Visual tracking and the primate flocculus.* Science 189:1000, 1975.

23. HIKOSAKA, D, AND MAEDA, M: *Cervical effects on abducens motoneurons and their interaction with vestibulo-ocular reflex.* Exp Brain Res 18:512, 1973.

24. DEJONG, PTVM, DEJONG, JMBV, COHEN, B, AND JONGKEES, LBW: *Ataxia and nystagmus induced by injection of local anesthetics in the neck.* Ann Neurol 1:240, 1977.

25. BRODAL, A: *Anatomy of the vestibular nuclei and their connections.* In KORNHUBER, HH (ED): *Handbook of Sensory Physiology, vol. VI, part I.* Springer-Verlag, New York, 1974.

26. BRODAL, A: *Anatomical organization of cerebello-vestibulo-spinal pathways.* In DE RENCK, AVS, AND KNIGHT, J (EDS): *Ciba Foundation Symposium:*

Myotatic, kinesthetic and vestibular mechanisms. Churchill Ltd, London, 1967.

27. POMPEIANO, O: *Cerebello-vestibular interrelations.* In KORNHUBER, HH (ED) *Handbook of Sensory Physiology. The Vestibular System, vol. VI, part 1.* Springer-Verlag, New York, 1974.

28. MCNALLY, WJ, AND STUART, EA: *Physiology of the Labyrinth. A manual prepared for graduates in medicine.* Am Acad Ophthalmol Otolaryngol, McGill University and Royal Victoria Hospital, Montreal, 1967.

29. HAWRYLSHYN, PA, RUBIN, AM, TASKER, RR, et al.: *Vestibulothalamic projections in man, a sixth primary sensory pathway.* J Neurophysiol 41:394, 1978.

30. ODKVIST, LM, LIEDGREN, SRC, AND ASCHAN, G: *Cerebral cortex and vestibular nerve.* Adv Oto-Rhino-Laryngol. 22:125, 1977.

31. PENFIELD, W: *Vestibular-sensation and the cerebral cortex.* Ann Otol Rhino Laryngol 66:691, 1957.

32. GACEK, R, LYON, M: *The localization of vestibular efferent neurons in the kitten with horseradish peroxidase.* Acta Otolaryngol (Stockh) 77:92, 1974.

33. WILSON, VJ, MELVILL JONES, G: *Mammalian Vestibular Physiology.* Plenum Press, New York, 1979.

34. GOLDBERG, JM, FERNANDEZ, C: *Efferent vestibular system in the squirrel monkey: Anatomical location and influence on afferent activity.* J. Neurophysiol 43:986, 1980.

35. BRICOUT-BERTHOUT A, AND CASTON, J: *Responses of afferent and efferent neurons to auditory inputs in the vestibular nerve of the frog.* J Comp Physiol Psychol 147:305, 1982.

4

THE CENTRAL
AUDITORY SYSTEM

THE COCHLEAR NUCLEI

OTHER PONTINE NUCLEI AND PATHWAYS

THE STAPEDIUS REFLEX

INFERIOR COLLICULUS
   AND MEDIAL GENICULATE BODY

THE AUDITORY CORTEX

THE AUDITORY EFFERENT SYSTEM

THE COCHLEAR NUCLEI

At the surface of the brain the cochlear nucleus can be seen as a swelling of the cochlear nerve as it enters the dorsolateral brainstem at the junction of the pons and medulla. The nucleus curves upward and medially over the restiform body and is covered superolaterally by the middle cerebellar peduncle. Two major subdivisions are generally recognized: the dorsal cochlear nucleus and the ventral cochlear nucleus.

Upon entering the brainstem the primary auditory afferent fibers divide into two branches, an anterior branch that terminates in the anterior part of the ventral cochlear nucleus, and a longer posterior branch that further divides, with one branch ending in the posterior part of the ventral cochlear nucleus, and the other terminating in the dorsal cochlear nucleus (Fig. 21).[1] Primary cochlear neurons do not bypass or send collaterals beyond the cochlear nucleus.[2] The orderly spatial arrangement present in the cochlea and cochlear nerve is main-

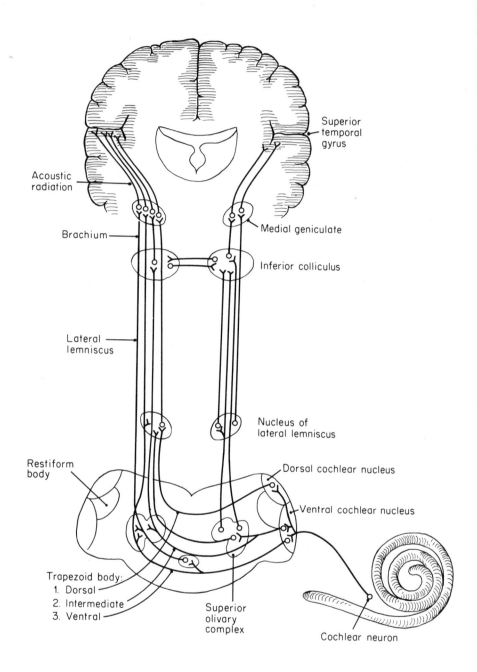

FIGURE 21. Central auditory pathways.

tained in the ventral cochlear nucleus. Axons that originate from cochlear neurons at the basal end of the cochlea terminate in the most medial and rostral areas of the ventral cochlear nucleus, while axons originating from neurons in the apex terminate on secondary neurons in the lateral caudal area of the ventral cochlear nucleus.[1]

Neurons in the dorsal cochlear nucleus send their axons into the dorsal trapezoid body, where they cross the midline and ascend in the contralateral lateral lemniscus. The cell bodies of the ventral cochlear nucleus send axons in the ventral trapezoid body to the ipsilateral and contralateral superior olivary complex. Some of the latter fibers synapse, and others traverse the superior olivary complex and run in the contralateral lateral lemniscus to the inferior colliculus and medial geniculate body.

OTHER PONTINE NUCLEI AND PATHWAYS

Nearly all axons leaving the cochlear nucleus synapse at least once in cell groups between the pontomedullary junction and the midbrain.[3] Three pontine nuclear groups can be identified: the trapezoid nucleus, the superior olivary complex, and the nucleus of the lateral lemniscus (see Fig. 21). The trapezoid nucleus receives input from the ventral cochlear nucleus on one side and projects to the lateral lemniscus of the opposite side. The superior olivary complex receives input from the ipsilateral and contralateral ventral cochlear nucleus, and projects to the nucleus of the lateral lemniscus and the inferior colliculus. The nucleus of the lateral lemniscus receives input from the dorsal and ventral cochlear nucleus, the trapezoid nucleus, and the superior olivary complex, and projects to the inferior colliculus and medial geniculate body.

These pontine nuclei function as relay stations for ascending auditory signals and as reflex centers. They represent the first anatomic location where binaural integration of auditory signals occurs consequent to crossing of a roughly equal proportion of afferent auditory fibers. Unilateral hearing loss cannot result from injury to these and the more rostral auditory nuclear groups.

THE STAPEDIUS REFLEX

A clinically important auditory reflex is the acoustic or stapedius reflex (Fig. 22).[4,5] The stapedius muscle contracts bilaterally in response to sound intensities of 70 to 90 dB above threshold hearing. The reflex activity is maintained for the duration of the stimulus. The stapedius reflex appears to be a protective mechanism to limit the movement of the sound transmitting system in the presence of high intensity sound. This is not the only function of the reflex, however, since it is also activated by low intensity sound pressure levels. The stapedius reflex may act in the processing of speech, since patients with stapedius paralysis due to Bell's palsy have impaired ability to discriminate speech.[5]

The reflex arc consists of (1) the hair cells in the organ of Corti, (2) primary afferent auditory neurons, (3) ipsilateral secondary neurons in the ventral cochlear nucleus, (4) bilateral tertiary neurons in the superior olivary nucleus, and (5)

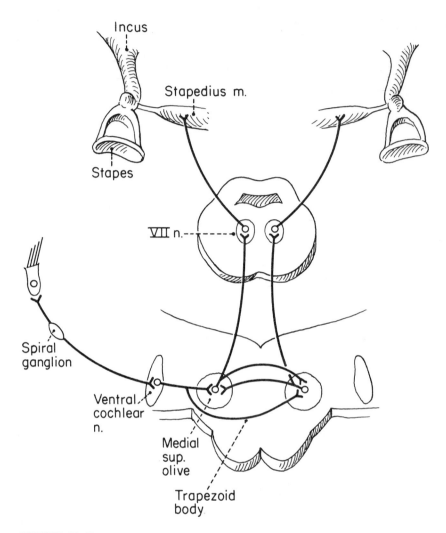

Incus

Stapedius m.

Stapes

VII n.

Spiral
ganglion

Ventral
cochlear
n.

Medial
sup.
olive

Trapezoid
body

FIGURE 22. The acoustic reflex. Schematic drawing of the direct excitatory connections from the cochlea to the stapedius muscle. (From Baloh, RW: *Neurotology.* In: *Clinical Neurology.* Baker, AB and Baker, LH (eds). JB Lippincott, Philadelphia, 1983, with permission).

bilateral stapedius motor neurons in the facial nucleus (Fig. 22). As with the canal-ocular reflex, a parallel multisynaptic pathway from the cochlear nucleus to stapedius motor neurons also exists. If the middle ear structures are intact, loss of the stapedius reflex indicates a lesion of (1) the auditory nerve, (2) the pons, or (3) the facial nerve (see Impedance Audiometry, Chapter 8).

INFERIOR COLLICULUS
AND MEDIAL GENICULATE BODY

The inferior colliculi are two rounded elevations forming the caudal half of the midbrain tectal plate. The main projection of the inferior colliculus is to the ipsilateral medial geniculate body via the brachium of the inferior colliculus (see Fig. 21). The medial geniculate bodies are small rounded elevations on the posterior aspect of each thalamus. No axon of a secondary cochlear neuron reaches the medial geniculate without first synapsing in one of the pontine nuclei or the inferior colliculus, and no ascending neuron bypasses the medial geniculate body.[6] The colliculi have numerous crossover connections as well as rich connections with the nearby reticular formation. There are no commissural connections between the medial geniculate bodies.

THE AUDITORY CORTEX

The auditory cortex in man is located in the superior temporal gyrus along the sylvian fissure (see Fig. 21).[3,7] By Brodmann's classification it corresponds to areas 41, 42, and 22.

Each sensory modality has a primary cortical reception area surrounded by association areas where integration of primary signals occurs. The primary auditory reception area, Brodmann's area 41, receives its projection from the rostral portion of the pars principalis of the medial geniculate body. An orderly spatial arrangement of tones has been demonstrated in the spiral ganglion of the cochlea, the cochlear nerve trunk, the ventral cochlear nucleus, the superior olivary nucleus, the rostral portions of the medial geniculate body, and the primary auditory cortex.[3,6] In the primary auditory cortex high frequencies are represented anteriorly, and low frequencies posteriorly. Areas 42 and 22, immediately adjacent to the primary auditory cortex, are auditory association areas. These areas receive signals from the primary reception area and project to regions of the occipital, parietal, and insular cortex.

In man, electrical stimulation close to the margins of the sylvian fissure in the area of the primary auditory cortex produces a sensation of simple sounds, such as a buzzing or ringing, while stimulation away from the fissure, in the association areas, introduces an element of interpretation to the sound, such as a dog barking or a familiar voice.[8] The further the stimulating electrode moves from the primary reception area, the more complex the interpretation (i.e., the higher the level of integration).

Because of the bilateral representation of hearing at the cortical level, hemispherectomy has no effect on hearing as judged by the pure tone audiogram.[9] However, such patients do have impaired discrimination of distorted, interrupted, or accelerated speech, particularly when presented to the contralateral ear (see Central Auditory Speech Tests, Chapter 8). Deficits in the production and comprehension of language (aphasia) complicate the clinical analysis of hearing in patients with bilateral lesions of the auditory cortex. However, a few cases have been reported in which bilateral cerebral lesions produce severe hearing loss in all spheres, and not simply an inability to understand spoken language.[10] Recent improvement in our ability to image the brain should lead to better clinical-pathological correlation in such patients.

THE AUDITORY EFFERENT SYSTEM

A large number of descending neurons parallel the ascending pathways (outlined in preceding sections) and link the auditory cortex with the lower auditory centers.[11] The main efferent pathway to the organ of Corti, the olivocochlear bundle, originates in the superior olivary complex on both sides, approximately 75 percent of fibers from the contralateral, and 25 percent from the ipsilateral superior olivary complex.[12] The fibers from both sides join the vestibular nerve root just beyond the genu of the facial nerve, then send collaterals to the ventral cochlear nucleus as the nerve passes directly beneath it. The auditory efferent fibers emerge from the brainstem in the inferior division of the vestibular nerve and follow this nerve to the cochlea, where they eventually end on afferent nerve endings at the base of the hair cells.

The specific function of the auditory efferent system is yet to be defined. The widespread branching of each efferent nerve fiber makes it unlikely that they have a localized effect on specific parts of the cochlea.[12] Stimulation of the olivocochlear bundle results in suppression of auditory nerve activity, but sectioning the bundle does not alter behavioral auditory function in the cat.[13,14] Furthermore, pure tone hearing levels are not affected in patients who have undergone vestibular nerve sectioning for chronic recurrent vertigo. The efferent auditory system may be involved in such behavioral phenomena as attention, frequency discrimination, or detection of signal in noise.

REFERENCES

1. SANDO, I: *The anatomical interrelationships of the cochlea nerve fibers.* Acta Otolaryngol (Stockh) 59:417, 1965.

2. LORENTE DE No, R: *Central representation of the eight nerve.* In GOODHILL, V (ED): *Ear Diseases, Deafness and Dizziness.* Harper and Row, Hagerstown, MD, 1979.

3. DUBLIN, WB: *Fundamentals of Sensorineural Auditory Pathology.* CC Thomas, Springfield, IL, 1976.

4. BORG, E: *On the neuronal organization of the acoustic middle ear reflex. A physiological and anatomical study.* Brain Res 49:101, 1973.

5. ZAKRISSON, J, BORG, E, AND BLOM, S: *The acoustic impedance charge as a measure of stapedius muscle activity in man.* Acta Otolaryngol (Stockh) 78:357, 1974.

6. SCHUKNECHT, HF: *Pathology of the Ear.* Harvard University Press, Cambridge, MA, 1974.

7. WOOLSEY, CN: *Organization of cortical auditory system: A review and synthesis.* In RASMUSSEN, GL, AND WINDLE, WF (EDS): *Neural Mechanisms of the Auditory and Vestibular Systems.* CC Thomas, Springfield, IL, 1960.

8. PENFIELD, W, AND JASPER, H: *Epilepsy and the Functional Anatomy of the Human Brain.* Little, Brown and Co, Boston, 1954.

9. DIX, MR, AND HOOD, JD: *Symmetrical hearing loss in brain stem lesions.* Acta Otolaryngol (Stockh) 75:165, 1973.

10. GRAHAM, J, GREENWOOD, R, AND LECKY, B: *Cortical deafness. A case report and review of the literature.* J Neurol Sci 48:35, 1980.

11. RASMUSSEN, GL: *Anatomical relationships of the ascending and descending auditory systems.* In RASMUSSEN, GL, AND WINDLE, WF (EDS): *Neural Mechanisms of the Auditory and Vestibular Pathways.* CC Thomas, Springfield, IL, 1960.

12. RASMUSSEN, GL: *Efferent connection of the cochlear nucleus.* In GRAHAM, AB (ED): *Sensorineural Hearing Processes and Disorders.* Little, Brown and Co, Boston, 1967.

13. GALAMBOS, R: *Suppression of auditory nerve activity by stimulation of efferent fibers to cochlea.* J Neurophysiol 19:424, 1956.

14. IGARASHI, M, ALFORD, BR, NAKAI, Y, et al: *Behavioral auditory function after transection of crossed olivo-cochlear bundle in the cat.* Acta Otolaryngol (Stockh) 73:455, 1972.

PART 2
HISTORY AND EXAMINATION

5

VESTIBULAR SYMPTOMS

DIZZINESS

IMBALANCE

VISUAL DISTORTION

SEVERITY OF SYMPTOMS

ASSOCIATED SYMPTOMS

MOTION SICKNESS

As described in preceding sections, the function of the vestibular system is to transduce the forces associated with head acceleration and gravity into a biologic signal that the brain can use to develop a subjective awareness of head position in space (orientation) and to produce motor reflexes for postural and ocular stability. Not surprisingly, lesions of the vestibular system commonly result in a sense of disorientation (dizziness), postural and gait imbalance, and visual distortion.

DIZZINESS

Since visual, proprioceptive, and vestibular signals provide critical information about the position of the head and body in space, damage to any of these systems can lead to a complaint of dizziness.[1] However, certain features in the patient's description of the dizziness can help the examining physician determine if the vestibular system is involved (Fig. 23).

An illusion of movement is specific for vestibular system disease. The most common illusion is that of rotation (vertigo), although patients occasionally complain of linear displacement or tilt. The afferent nerves from the otoliths and

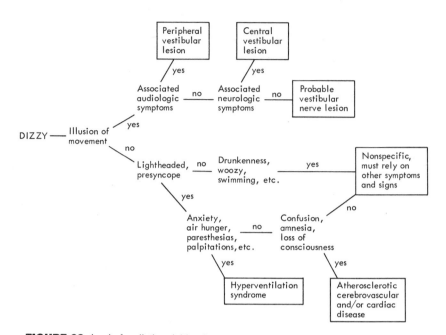

FIGURE 23. Logic for distinguishing between different causes of dizziness.

semicircular canals of each labyrinth maintain a balanced tonic rate of firing into the vestibular nuclei. Asymmetric involvement of this baseline activity leads to a sensation of movement. For example, damage to a semicircular canal or its afferent nerve produces a sensation of angular rotation in the plane of that canal. More commonly, lesions involve all the canals and otoliths of one labyrinth, producing a sensation of rotation in a plane determined by the balance of afferent signals from the contralateral labyrinth (usually near the horizontal, since the vertical canal and otolith signals partially cancel out). If a patient with such a lesion attempts to fixate on an object, it will appear blurred and seem to be moving in the opposite direction of the slow phase of his spontaneous nystagmus (i.e., away from the side of the lesion). This illusion of movement occurs because the brain lacks eye proprioceptive information, and interprets the target displacement on the retina as object movement rather than eye movement. By contrast, if the patient closes his eyes he senses that his body is turning toward the side of the lesion, owing to the imbalance of tonic vestibular signals arriving at the subjective sensation centers of the cortex. An illusion of linear movement alone suggests isolated involvement of an otolith or its central connections.

Although an illusion of movement always indicates an imbalance in the vestibular system (including visual-vestibular and nuchal-vestibular pathways), its absence does not rule out a vestibular lesion. Other descriptions of the sensation associated with vestibular dysfunction include giddiness, swimming in the head, floating, and drunkenness. Symptoms of autonomic dysfunction, (e.g., sweating, pallor, nausea, and vomiting) nearly always accompany dizziness caused by vestibular lesions. Occasionally, vegetative symptoms are the only manifestation of such a lesion. Numerous interconnecting pathways between brainstem vestibular and autonomic centers account for this close association of vestibular and autonomic symptoms.

A presyncopal light-headed sensation is rarely, if ever, produced by vestibular lesions. This type of dizziness is most commonly associated with diffuse cerebral ischemia. In young patients it typically occurs with chronic anxiety and hyperventilation. Associated symptoms include frequent sighing, air hunger, perioral numbness, paresthesias of the extremities, lump in throat, palpitations, and tightness of the chest.[2] Hyperventilation causes dizziness by lowering carbon dioxide content of the blood, producing constriction of the cerebral vasculature.[3] In older patients presyncopal light-headedness typically results from diffuse atherosclerotic cerebrovascular disease along with decreased cardiac output. Postural hypotension and transient cardiac arrhythmias are common precipitating factors for this type of dizziness.

Some patients complain of dizziness when they first wear glasses, experiencing a vague feeling of disorientation often accompanied by headache. Dizziness most frequently accompanies correction of astigmatism, but also occurs after a change in magnification. Elderly patients who undergo cataract surgery may experience severe dizziness when first fitted with new lenses. A dizzy sensation is commonly produced by imbalance in the extraocular muscles. After an acute ocular muscle paralysis, looking in the direction of the paralyzed muscles causes dizziness (in addition to diplopia), but within a short time the nervous system adapts to the altered spatial information. Dizziness associated with visual defects is rarely severe and an illusion of movement does not occur.

Not infrequently, one can trace dizziness to lesions involving multiple sensory systems, particularly in elderly patients, or in patients with systemic disorders such as diabetes mellitus.[4] A typical combination might include peripheral neuropathy resulting in diminished touch and proprioceptive input, decreased visual acuity (cataracts, glaucoma), and impaired hearing (as with presbycusis). In such patients an added vestibular impairment (from ototoxic drugs, for example) can be devastating, making it impossible for them to walk without assistance. Patients with multisensory dizziness do poorly in unfamiliar surroundings; they are unable to adapt because of their impaired sensory input.

Events just prior to an episode of dizziness are important in determining the cause. Dizziness caused by vestibular lesions is usually worsened by rapid head movements, since the new stimulus is sensed by the intact labyrinth, and existing asymmetries are accentuated. Episodes may be precipitated by turning over in bed, sitting up from the lying position, extending the neck to look up, or bending over and straightening up. Patients with a perilymph fistula have brief episodes of vertigo precipitated by changes in middle ear pressure (coughing, sneezing). The pressure change in the middle ear is transferred directly to the inner ear (usually the horizontal semicircular canal) through the bony fistula.

Occasionally, loud noises induce transient dizziness in patients with Meniere's syndrome (Tulio phenomenon). As the labyrinthine membranes dilate owing to increased endolymphatic pressure, adhesions may develop between the stapedius footplate and the membranous labyrinth, resulting in traction on the sensory receptors with sudden movement of the stapes (see Fig. 59).

The nervous system has a remarkable ability to compensate for an imbalance within the vestibular system, and thus dizziness due to vestibular lesions usually occurs in episodes. Of the commonly encountered vestibular syndromes, brief episodes lasting only seconds are typical of so-called benign paroxysmal positional vertigo. Episodes lasting minutes are characteristic of vascular syndromes, such as transient vertebrobasilar insufficiency and migraine. Vertigo during a typical bout of Meniere's syndrome lasts for 3 to 4 hours, although the patient often complains of a vague sense of dizziness for a day or so thereafter. Viral labyrinthitis and mononeuritis of the vestibular nerve are characterized by the acute onset of severe vertigo, followed by gradual decreasing intensity over several days. Continuous dizziness without fluctuation for long periods of time is not typical of peripheral vestibular disorders.

IMBALANCE

With acute unilateral vestibular lesions, asymmetry of tonic vestibulospinal activity leads to postural and gait imbalance, with a tendency for the patient to fall toward the side of the lesion. This gait unsteadiness is rapidly compensated for, usually lasting less than a week. Patients with a slowly progressive unilateral lesion may not experience any imbalance. Bilateral symmetrical vestibular loss results in a more pronounced and persistent unsteadiness that may be incapacitating in elderly patients. This is particularly likely if the patient has other sensory deficits, such as peripheral neuropathy and impaired vision (multisensory dizziness). The imbalance due to loss of vestibulospinal function is typically worse at night when the patient is less able to use vision to compensate for the vestibular loss. The flow chart in Figure 24 summarizes the logic for distinguishing between imbalance due to vestibular lesions and that due to cerebellar and proprioceptive lesions.

VISUAL DISTORTION

Different types of visual distortion can result from lesions of the vestibulo-ocular pathways. If the patient attempts to fixate on an object after an acute unilateral peripheral vestibular lesion, it will appear blurred and seem to be moving in the opposite direction of the slow phase of his spontaneous nystagmus. Oscillopsia associated with unilateral peripheral vestibular lesions is usually transient, disappearing as the acute vertigo and spontaneous nystagmus disappear. Occasionally, such patients will have persistent head movement dependent oscillopsia, probably due to inadequate central compensation for the peripheral loss.

Patients with bilateral symmetrical loss of vestibular function develop oscillopsia with any head movement.[1,5] Characteristically, when walking they are

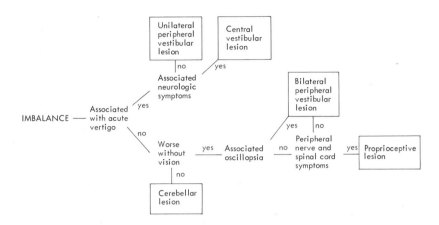

FIGURE 24. Logic for distinguishing between different causes of imbalance.

unable to fixate on objects because the surroundings are bouncing up and down. In order to see the faces of passersby they learn to stop and hold their head still (or to say hello to all indiscriminately). When reading, such patients learn to place their hand on their chin to prevent slight movements associated with pulsatile cerebral blood flow. Patients with spontaneous nystagmus due to lesions of the central vestibulo-ocular pathways also report oscillopsia, but in this case the oscillopsia is constant, and usually associated with other neurologic symptoms. The flow chart in Figure 25 outlines how one distinguishes between the different causes of oscillopsia based on the clinical history.

SEVERITY OF SYMPTOMS

The severity of symptoms following a vestibular lesion depends on (1) the extent of the lesion, (2) whether the lesion is unilateral or bilateral, and (3) the rapidity with which the functional loss occurs. Patients who slowly lose vestibular function bilaterally (for example, secondary to ototoxic drugs) often do not complain of dizziness, but will report oscillopsia with head movements and instability when walking (owing to loss of vestibulo-ocular and vestibulo-spinal reflex activity respectively). If a patient slowly loses vestibular function on one side only over a period of months to years (for example, with an acoustic neuroma), symptoms and signs may be absent. On the other hand, a sudden unilateral loss of vestibular function is a dramatic event. The patient complains of severe dizziness and nausea, and is pale and perspiring and usually vomits repeatedly. He prefers to lie quietly in a dark room, but can walk if forced to (falling toward the side of the lesion). A brisk spontaneous nystagmus interferes with vision. These symptoms and signs are transient, and the process of compensation begins almost immediately. Within one week of the lesion a young patient can walk without difficulty and, with fixation, can inhibit the spontaneous nys-

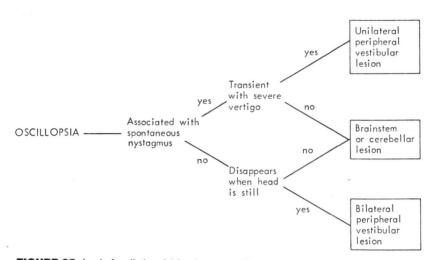

FIGURE 25. Logic for distinguishing between different causes of oscillopsia.

tagmus. Within one month most patients return to work with little, if any, residual symptoms.

ASSOCIATED SYMPTOMS

Unfortunately, the description of vestibular symptoms does not differentiate peripheral from central lesions. For this, one must rely on the associated symptoms. Lesions of the labyrinth or VIIIth nerve usually produce auditory symptoms such as hearing loss, tinnitus, a sensation of pressure or fullness in the ear, and pain in the ear. In addition to hearing loss and tinnitus, lesions of the internal auditory canal are often associated with ipsilateral facial weakness, while those in the cerebellopontine angle may have ipsilateral facial numbness and weakness and ipsilateral extremity ataxia.

Because of the close approximation of other neuronal centers and fiber tracts in the brainstem and cerebellum, it is unusual to find lesions in these areas that produce isolated vestibular symptoms. Lesions of the brainstem invariably are associated with other cranial nerve and long tract symptoms. For example, vertigo caused by transient vertebrobasilar insufficiency is associated with other brainstem and occipital lobe symptoms such as diplopia, hemianoptic field defects, drop attacks, weakness, numbness, dysarthria, and ataxia. Lesions of the cerebellum (e.g., infarction or hemorrhage) may be relatively silent, but are always associated with extremity and truncal ataxia in addition to vertigo. Of note, hearing loss for pure tones is unusual with brainstem lesions, even in the late stages.

Vertigo can occur as part of an aura of temporal lobe seizures. The cortical projections of the vestibular system are activated by a focal discharge within the temporal lobe. Such vertigo is nearly always associated with other typical aura symptoms, such as an abnormal taste or smell and distortion of the visual world (hallucinations and illusions). Occasionally, however, vertigo can be the only manifestation of an aura. In such cases the association with typical "absence" spells should lead one to the correct diagnosis.

MOTION SICKNESS

Motion sickness refers to the syndrome of dizziness, perspiration, nausea, vomiting, increased salivation, yawning, and generalized malaise caused by excessive stimulation of the vestibular system.[6,7] Although it is usually produced by prolonged stimulation of the labyrinthine end organs, persistent visual stimulation with an optokinetic drum can also produce the syndrome.[8] Both linear and angular head acceleration induce motion sickness if applied for prolonged periods in susceptible subjects. Combinations of linear and angular acceleration, or multiplanar angular accelerations, are particularly effective. Rotation about the vertical axis, along with either voluntary or involuntary nodding movements in the sagittal plane, rapidly produce motion sickness in nearly everybody. This movement combines linear and angular acceleration (Coriolis effect).

Autonomic symptoms are usually the initial manifestation of motion sickness.[7] Sensitive sweat detectors can identify increased sweating as soon as 5 seconds after onset of motion, and grossly detectable sweating is usually apparent before any noticeable nausea. Increased salivation and frequent swallowing movements occur. Gastric motility is reduced and digestion is impaired. Hyperventilation is almost always present, and the resulting hypocapnia leads to changes in blood volume with pooling in the lower parts of the body, predisposing the subject to postural hypotension. Motion sickness effects the appetite, so that even the sight or smell of food is distressing.

Patients with nonfunctioning labyrinths are immune to motion sickness under all test conditions, even after prolonged exposure to wave motion during a storm at sea in which all sensory modalities are vigorously stimulated.[7] Some normal subjects are sensitive to development of motion sickness, while others are highly resistant. Unfortunately, there is no reliable way to predict who will develop motion sickness.[9] Most subjects will eventually adapt to prolonged vestibular stimulation, but some never completely adapt (the chronically seasick ocean voyager). An unusual variant of motion sickness is the mal de debarquement syndrome. In this case motion sickness continues when the subject returns to stationary conditions after prolonged exposure to motion. Typically, patients report that they feel the persistent rocking sensation of the boat long after returning to dry land. This syndrome can last for months to years after the exposure to motion, and occasionally is incapacitating. The cause of the mal de debarquement syndrome is unknown.

REFERENCES

1. BALOH, RW, AND HONRUBIA, V: *Clinical Neurophysiology of the Vestibular System.* FA Davis, Philadelphia, 1979.

2. SINGER, EP: *The hyperventilation syndrome in clinical medicine.* New York J Med 58:1494, 1958.

3. GOTCH, F, MEYER, JS, AND YASUYUKI, T: *Cerebral effects of hyperventilation in man.* Arch Neurol 12:410, 1965.

4. DRACHMAN, DA, AND HART, CW: *An approach to the dizzy patient.* Neurology 22:323, 1972.

5. HESS, K, GRESTY, M, AND LEECH, J: *Clinical and theoretical aspects of head movement dependent oscillopsia (HMDO). A review.* J Neurol 219:151, 1978.

6. MONEY, KE: *Motion sickness.* Physiol Rev 50:1, 1970.

7. JOHNSON, WH, AND JONGKEES, LBW: *Motion sickness.* In KORNHUBER, HH (ED): *Handbook of Sensory Physiology, vol VI, part 2.* Springer-Verlag, New York, 1974.

8. DICHGANS, J, AND BRANDT, T: *Visual-vestibular integration and motion perception.* In BIZZI, E, AND DICHGANS, F (EDS): *Cerebral Control of Eye Movements and Motion Perception.* S Karger, Basel, 1972.

9. JONKEES, LBW: *Motion sickness. II. Some sensory aspects.* In KORNHUBER, HH (ED): *Handbook of Sensory Physiology, vol. VI, part 2.* Springer-Verlag, New York, 1974.

6

AUDITORY SYMPTOMS

HEARING LOSS
   Conductive
   Sensorineural
   Central
TINNITUS
   Objective
   Subjective

The main symptoms of lesions within the auditory system are hearing loss and tinnitus.[1,2] Hearing loss can be classified as conductive, sensorineural, and central, based on the anatomic site of pathology. Tinnitus can be either subjective or objective.

HEARING LOSS

Conductive

Conductive hearing loss results from lesions involving the external or middle ear. The tympanic membrane and ossicles act as a transformer, amplifying airborne sound and efficiently transferring it to the inner ear fluid. If this normal pathway is obstructed, transmission can occur across the skin and through the bones of the skull (bone conduction), but at the cost of significant energy loss. Patients with a conductive hearing loss can hear speech in a noisy background better than in a quiet background, since they can understand loud speech as well as anyone.

     The most common cause of conductive hearing loss is impacted cerumen in the external canal. This benign condition is often first noticed after bathing or swimming, when a droplet of water closes the remaining tiny passageway. The most common serious cause of conductive hearing loss is inflammation of the middle ear, otitis media.[3] Either infected (suppurative otitis) or noninfected (serous otitis) fluid accumulates in the middle ear, impairing the conduction of airborne sound. With chronic otitis media, a cholesteatoma may erode the ossicles. Otosclerosis produces progressive conductive hearing loss by immobilizing the stapes with new bone growth in front of and below the oval window. Other common causes of conductive hearing loss include trauma, congenital malformations of the external and middle ear, and glomus body tumors.

Sensorineural

Sensorineural hearing loss results from lesions of the cochlea or the auditory division of the VIII cranial nerve, or both. The spiral cochlea mechanically analyzes the frequency content of sound. For high frequency tones, only sensory cells in the basilar turn are activated, while for low frequency ones all, or nearly all, sensory cells are activated. Therefore, with lesions of the cochlea and its afferent nerve, the hearing levels for different frequencies are usually unequal and the phase relationship (timing) between different frequencies may be altered. Patients with sensorineural hearing loss often have difficulty hearing speech that is mixed with background noise, and may be annoyed by loud speech.

Distortion of sounds is common with sensorineural hearing loss. A pure tone may be heard as noisy, rough, or buzzing, or it may be distorted so that it sounds like a complex mixture of tones. Binaural diplacusis occurs when the two ears are affected unequally, so that the same frequency has a different pitch in each ear, that is, the patient hears double. Monaural diplacusis occurs when two tones, or a tone and noise, are heard simultaneously in one ear. With recruitment there is an abnormally rapid growth in the sensation of loudness as the intensity of a sound is increased, so that faint or moderate sounds cannot be heard, while there is little or no change in the loudness of loud sounds.

The most common cause of *sudden* unilateral sensorineural hearing loss is infection of the inner ear (labyrinthitis).[4] Bacteria can enter the inner ear directly from the middle ear, or from the cerebrospinal fluid via the cochlear aqueduct and internal auditory canal. In the former case, there is a history of recurrent or chronic otitis media; in the latter case, the patient has bacterial meningitis. Viral labyrinthitis may be part of a systemic viral illness, such as measles, mumps, and infectious mononucleosis, or an isolated infection of the labyrinth without systemic symptoms. Mumps is a particularly common cause of unilateral hearing loss in preschool and school-aged children. Other common causes of acute unilateral hearing loss are head trauma and vascular occlusive disease.

Relapsing unilateral sensorineural hearing loss associated with tinnitus, ear fullness, and vertigo is typical of Meniere's syndrome. Ototoxic drugs produce a bilateral *subacute* hearing loss. Acoustic neuromas (vestibular schwannomas) characteristically produce a *slowly progressive* unilateral sensorineural hearing loss. The *chronic progressive* bilateral hearing loss associated with advancing age is called presbycusis. It may include conductive and central dysfunction, but the most consistent effect of aging is on the sensory cells and neurons of the cochlea.

Central

Central hearing disorders result from lesions of the central auditory pathways. As described in Chapter 4, these consist of the cochlear and dorsal olivary nuclear complexes, inferior colliculi, medial geniculate bodies, auditory cortex in the temporal lobes, and interconnecting afferent and efferent fiber tracts. As a rule, patients with central lesions do not have impaired hearing levels for pure tones, and they understand speech as long as it is clearly spoken in a quiet environment. If the listener's task is made more difficult with the introduction of background or competing messages, performance deteriorates more markedly in patients with central lesions than in normal subjects (see Central Auditory Speech Tests, Chapter 8). Lesions involving the VIII nerve root entry zone or cochlear nucleus, however, can result in unilateral hearing loss for pure tones (e.g., demyelination or infarction in the lateral pontomedullary region). Since approximately 50 percent of afferent nerve fibers cross central to the cochlear nucleus, this is the most central structure in which a lesion can result in a unilateral hearing loss.

TINNITUS

Tinnitus is a noise or ringing in the ear that is usually audible only to the patient, although rarely the sound can be heard by an examiner as well as the patient (so-called objective tinnitus.)[5,6] The flow chart in Figure 26 summarizes the logic for distinguishing between different causes of tinnitus.

Objective

Objective tinnitus can be heard when the examining physician places a stethoscope into the patient's external auditory canal. A blowing sound that coincides with inspiration, expiration, or both, can result from an abnormally patent eustachian tube. This type of tinnitus commonly occurs after an extensive weight loss, or in patients with a debilitating illness. Tinnitus characterized by a series of sharp clicks heard for several seconds or minutes at a time can result from tetanic contractions of the muscles of the soft palate. These contractions can be observed by the examiner when the tinnitus is audible. Tinnitus that is pulsatory and synchronous with the heartbeat suggests a vascular abnormality within the head or neck. Aneurysms, arteriovenous malformations, and vascular tumors can produce this type of tinnitus. A venous hum can be either a continuous machine-like sound, or a "whoosh" in synchrony with the pulse. Light pressure on the neck that occludes the distal jugular vein, but not the arterial blood flow, stops the hum.[7] A venous hum is often associated with x-ray evidence of an

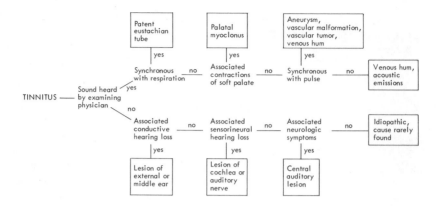

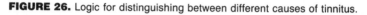

FIGURE 26. Logic for distinguishing between different causes of tinnitus.

enlarged jugular bulb, and ligation of the internal jugular vein can be curative in some patients.

Recently it has been shown that oscillatory vibrations within the cochlea can be heard in many normal ears when one uses a special ear canal recording technique.[8] These so-called acoustic emissions are audible to some subjects, and may be one source of mild tonal tinnitus, particularly in a quiet environment.

Subjective

Subjective tinnitus (heard only by the patient) can result from lesions involving the external ear canal, tympanic membrane, ossicles, cochlea, auditory nerve, brainstem, and cortex. The description of the noise can vary from an ill-defined buzzing, ringing, hissing, or whistling, to a more recognizable sound such as a cricket, seashell, or motor sound. The patient's description of the loudness, pitch, and duration of tinnitus can be diagnostically useful.[5] The characteristic tinnitus associated with Meniere's syndrome is low-pitched and continuous, typically described as an ocean roar or hollow seashell sound. Often the tinnitus becomes very loud immediately preceding an acute attack of vertigo, and then may transiently disappear after the attack. Tinnitus with otosclerosis is also usually low-pitched, described as a buzzing or roaring sound. It is usually continuous, but can occasionally be intermittent, or even pulsatile. In some patients with otosclerosis, the tinnitus is more disturbing than the hearing loss. A high-pitched ringing tinnitus is experienced in most subjects after a slap across the head, or close exposure to a sudden very loud noise, such as an explosion or the firing of a gun. This tinnitus usually subsides within a few hours, although occasionally, if permanent hearing loss has occurred from damage to the inner ear, a high-pitched ringing tinnitus may persist for years. Continuous bilateral high-pitched tinnitus often accompanies chronic noise-induced hearing loss, presbycusis, and hearing loss due to ototoxic drugs. Continuous unilateral high-pitched tinnitus may be the first symptom of an acoustic neuroma, preceding loss of hearing by several years.

As in the case of vertigo, the character of the tinnitus alone does not determine the site of the disturbance. For this, one must rely on associated symptoms and signs. When tinnitus results from a lesion of the external or middle ear, it is usually accompanied by a conductive hearing loss. The patient may complain that his voice sounds hollow and that other sounds are muffled. Since the masking effect of ambient noise is lost, the patient may be disturbed by normal muscular sounds such as chewing, tight closure of the eyes, or clenching of the jaws. Tinnitus caused by lesions of the cochlea or auditory nerve is usually associated with sensorineural hearing loss, distortion of sounds, or diplacusis, or both. The pitch of the tinnitus often corresponds to the frequency at which the hearing loss is greatest. Tinnitus resulting from lesions within the central nervous system is usually not associated with hearing loss, but is nearly always associated with other neurologic symptoms and signs.

As many as 50 percent of patients with tinnitus do not have associated hearing loss. In such patients the cause of the tinnitus is rarely identified. Numerous drugs can produce tinnitus without associated hearing loss.[9] Some of the more commonly used drugs include quinidine, salicylates, indomethacin, carbamazepine, propranolol, levodopa, aminophylline, and caffeine. The anatomic site of action of these drugs in producing tinnitus is unknown, although both peripheral and central effects probably occur. Many are known to affect biogenic amine neurotransmission within the central nervous system. Such drugs might produce tinnitus by facilitating or altering the balance of transmitted signals through the central auditory pathways. When cats are administered sodium salicylate to produce blood concentrations commonly associated with tinnitus in normal human subjects (0.3 to 0.6 mg per ml), the threshold of all primary afferent fibers is increased, irrespective of their characteristic frequency and spontaneous activity.[10] Associated with the increase in threshold is a reduction in the tuning and dynamic range of cochlear afferent fibers typical of the response to many other ototoxic drugs. However, with salicylates an increase in the spontaneous discharge rate occurs in those fibers whose spontaneous activity is greater than 20 spikes per second. This finding is an important exception to the general rule that depression of cochlear afferent nerve spontaneous activity occurs with damage to the cochlea.

REFERENCES

1. DAVIS, H, SILVERMAN, SR (EDS): *Hearing and Deafness, Ed 4.* Holt, Rinehart, and Winston, New York, 1978.
2. BEAGLEY, HA, (ED): *Audiology and Audiologic Medicine.* Oxford University Press, New York, 1981.
3. JAFFEE, BF (ED): *Hearing Loss in Children.* University Park Press, Baltimore, 1977.
4. SCHUKNECHT, HL: *Pathology of the Ear.* Harvard University Press, Cambridge, MA, 1974.

5. JACKSON, PD: In *Audiology and Audiologic Medicine.* Oxford University Press, New York, 1981.

6. DOUEK, E: *Classification of tinnitus.* In *CIBA Foundation Symposium No. 85,* London, 1981.

7. WARD, PH, BABIN, R, CALCATERRA, TC, AND KONRAD, HR: *Operative treatment of surgical lesions with objective tinnitus.* Ann Otol Rhinol Laryngol 84:473, 1975.

8. KEMP, DT: *Stimulated acoustic emissions from within the human auditory system.* J Acoust Soc Am 64:1386, 1978.

9. BROWN, D, PENNY, JE, HENLEY, CM, et al: *Ototoxic drugs and noise.* In *CIBA Foundation Symposium No. 85,* London, 1981.

10. EVANS, EF, WILSON, JP, AND BORERWE, TA: *Animal models of tinnitus.* In *CIBA Foundation Symposium No. 85,* London, 1981.

7

EXAMINATION OF
THE VESTIBULAR SYSTEM

BEDSIDE TESTS

Past Pointing

Past pointing refers to a reactive deviation of the extremities caused by an imbalance in the vestibular system. The test is performed by having the patient place his extended index finger on that of the examiner's, close his eyes, raise the extended arm and index finger to a vertical position, and attempt to return his index finger to the examiner's (Fig. 27). Consistent deviation to one side is past pointing. As with all tests of vestibulospinal function, extralabyrinthine influences should be eliminated as much as possible by having the patient seated with eyes closed and arm and index finger extended throughout the test. The standard finger-to-nose test will not identify past pointing, since joint and muscle proprioceptive signals permit accurate localization even when vestibular function is lost. Patients with acute peripheral vestibular damage past point toward the side of loss, but compensation usually corrects the past pointing, and can even produce a drift to the other side.[1]

Romberg Test

For the Romberg test (see Fig. 27) the patient stands with feet together, arms folded against the chest, and eyes closed. Patients with acute unilateral labyrinthine lesions sway and fall toward the damaged side. Like the past pointing test, however, the Romberg test is not a good indicator of chronic unilateral vestibular impairment, and sometimes the patient will fall toward the intact side.[1]

Tandem Walking

When performed with eyes open, tandem walking, or heel-to-toe walking (see Fig. 27), is primarily a test of cerebellar function, since vision compensates for chronic vestibular and proprioceptive deficits. Acute vestibular lesions, however, may impair tandem walking even with eyes open. Tandem walking with eyes closed provides a better test of vestibular function so long as cerebellar and proprioceptive function are intact. As with other tests of vestibulospinal function, however, the direction of falling in patients with chronic lesions is not a reliable indicator of the side of the lesion. So-called stepping or marching tests have the same limitation as the tandem walking test.[2]

The Doll's Eye Test

In an alert human, rotating the head back and forth in the horizontal plane induces compensatory horizontal eye movements that are dependent on both the fixation pursuit and vestibular systems. Because of the combined visual and vestibular input, a patient with complete loss of vestibular function and normal pursuit may still have normal compensatory eye movements on this test. The doll's eye test (see Fig. 27) is a useful bedside test of vestibular function in a

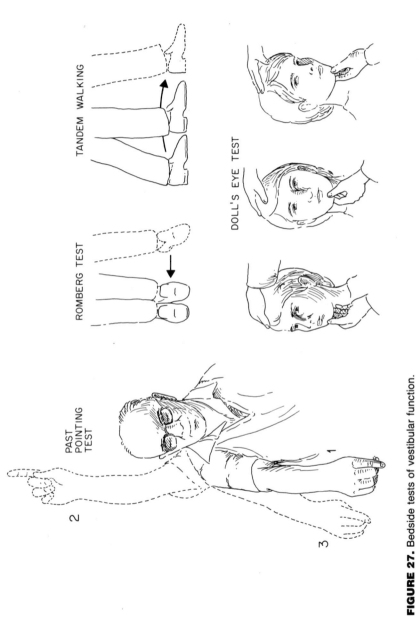

TANDEM WALKING

ROMBERG TEST

DOLL'S EYE TEST

PAST
POINTING
TEST

FIGURE 27. Bedside tests of vestibular function.

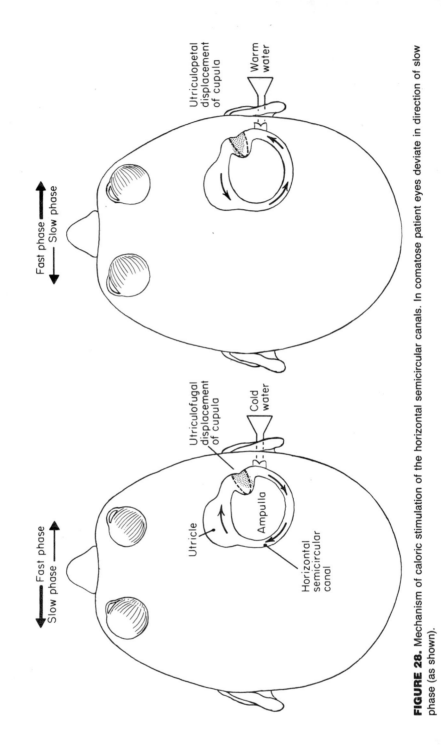

FIGURE 28. Mechanism of caloric stimulation of the horizontal semicircular canals. In comatose patient eyes deviate in direction of slow phase (as shown).

comatose patient, however, since such patients cannot generate pursuit or corrective fast components. In this setting, slow conjugate compensatory eye movements indicate normally functioning vestibulo-ocular pathways (i.e., those illustrated in Fig. 15).

Cold Caloric Test

The caloric test uses a nonphysiologic stimulus to induce endolymphatic flow in the horizontal semicircular canal, and thus horizontal nystagmus, by creating a temperature gradient from one side of the canal to the other.[1] With a cold caloric stimulus the column of endolymph nearest the middle ear falls because of its increased density. This causes the cupula to deviate away from the utricle (ampullofugal flow) and produces horizontal nystagmus with the fast phase directed away from the stimulated ear (Fig. 28). A warm stimulus produces the opposite effect, causing ampullopetal endolymph flow and nystagmus directed toward the stimulated ear (COWS—cold opposite, warm same). Because of its ready availability, iced water (approximately 0°C) is usually used for bedside caloric testing. To bring the horizontal canal into the vertical plane the patient lies in the supine position with the head tilted 30 degrees forward. Infusion of 10 ml of iced water induces a burst of nystagmus usually lasting from one to three minutes. In a comatose patient only a slow tonic deviation toward the side of stimulation is observed. In normal subjects the duration and speed of induced nystagmus varies greatly depending on the size of the external canal, the thickness of the temporal bone, the circulation to the temporal bone, and the subject's ability to use fixation to suppress the nystagmus.[3,4] Greater than a 20 percent asymmetry in nystagmus duration suggests a lesion on the side of the decreased response. This should always be confirmed, however, with standard bithermal caloric testing and electronystagmography (see below).

EVALUATION OF PATHOLOGIC NYSTAGMUS

Nystagmus is a nonvoluntary, rhythmic oscillation of the eyes that usually has a clearly defined fast and slow component. By convention the direction of the fast component defines the direction of nystagmus. Physiologic nystagmus refers to nystagmus that occurs in normal subjects, while pathologic nystagmus implies an underlying abnormality. Physiologic nystagmus may be vestibular induced (rotatory or caloric), visual induced (optokinetic), or may occur on extreme lateral gaze (end point). Pathologic nystagmus may be spontaneous (present in the primary position with the patient seated), positional (induced by a change in head position), or gaze-evoked (induced by a change in eye position). The flow charts in Figures 29, 31, and 33 summarize the logic for distinguishing between different varieties of pathologic nystagmus.

Spontaneous Nystagmus (Fig. 29)

A decrease in the baseline flow of action potentials from a single semicircular canal results in nystagmus in the plane of that canal with a slow conjugate

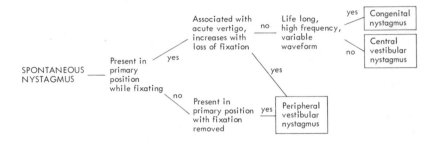

FIGURE 29. Logic for distinguishing between different types of spontaneous nystagmus.

deviation toward the damaged side interrupted by a quick corrective movement in the opposite direction (see Fig. 16). Since a selective loss of tonic afferent signals from one canal is unusual, *peripheral vestibular nystagmus* is usually rotatory because of the combined effects of altered vertical and horizontal canal input. The horizontal component is most prominent, however, because the components from the two vertical canals partially cancel each other. Gaze in the direction of the fast component increases the frequency and amplitude, while gaze in the opposite direction has the reverse effect (Alexander's law). Peripheral vestibular nystagmus (i.e., that resulting from lesions of the labyrinth or VIII nerve) is strongly inhibited by fixation. Unless the patient is seen within a few days of the acute episode, spontaneous nystagmus will not be present when fixation is permitted (i.e., on routine examination).[5] In this instance, Frenzel glasses (+ 20 lenses) are particularly useful for abolishing fixation and uncovering spontaneous vestibular nystagmus (Fig. 30). Acquired persistent spontaneous nystagmus that is not inhibited by fixation *(fixation nystagmus, central vestibular nystagmus)* indicates a lesion in the brainstem and/or cerebellum. Fixation nystagmus is often purely horizontal or vertical, since horizontal and vertical vestibular ocular pathways separate, beginning at the vestibular nuclei. Spontaneous *congenital nystagmus* is also prominent with fixation, but it can usually be distinguished from acquired fixation nystagmus based on its long duration, atypical waveforms (often pendular) and high frequency (usually 2 to 5 cps).

Positional Nystagmus (Fig. 31)

Two general types of positional nystagmus can be identified on the basis of nystagmus regularity: static and paroxysmal.[1,6] One induces static positional nystagmus by slowly placing the patient into the supine, right lateral, and left lateral positions. This type of positional nystagmus persists as long as the position is held. Paroxysmal positional nystagmus, on the other hand, is induced by a rapid change from erect sitting to the supine head-hanging left, center, or right

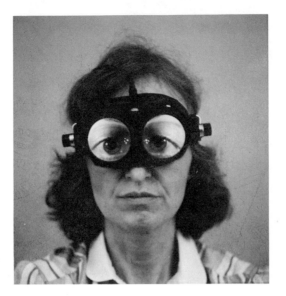

FIGURE 30. Frenzel glasses.

position. It is initially high in frequency, but rapidly dissipates within 30 seconds to a minute. The technique for performing rapid and slow positional testing is illustrated in Figure 32.

Static positional nystagmus often is not associated with vertigo and is seldom seen without the aid of Frenzel glasses to inhibit fixation. It may be unidirectional in all positions or direction-changing in different positions. Both direction-changing and direction-fixed static positional nystagmus occur most commonly with peripheral vestibular disorders, but both also occur with central lesions. Their presence only indicates a dysfunction in the vestibular system without localizing value. As with spontaneous nystagmus, however, lack of suppression with fixation and signs of associated brainstem dysfunction suggest a central lesion.

The most common variety of *paroxysmal positional nystagmus* (so-called benign paroxysmal positional nystagmus) usually has a 3 to 10 second latency before onset and rarely lasts longer than 15 seconds. The nystagmus is always torsional, with fast phase directed upward, that is, toward the forehead.[7] It is prominent in only one head-hanging position, and a burst of nystagmus in the reverse direction usually occurs when the patient moves back to the sitting position. Another key feature is that the patient experiences severe vertigo with initial positioning, but with repeated positioning vertigo and nystagmus rapidly disappear.

Benign paroxysmal positional nystagmus is a sign of vestibular end organ disease (see Degenerative Disorders of the Labyrinth, Chapter 9). It can be the

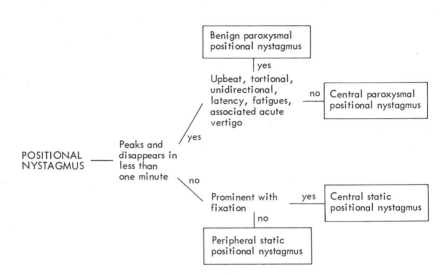

FIGURE 31. Logic for distinguishing between different types of positional nystagmus.

only finding in an otherwise healthy individual, or it may be associated with other signs of peripheral vestibular damage, such as vestibular nystagmus and unilateral caloric hypoexcitability.[7] In those instances where an abnormality is identified on caloric testing, the nystagmus invariably will occur when the patient is positioned with the damaged ear down. Benign paroxysmal positional nystagmus is a common sequella of head injury, viral labyrinthitis, and occlusion of the vasculature to the inner ear. In the majority of cases, however, it occurs as an isolated symptom of unknown cause.

Paroxysmal positional nystagmus can also result from brainstem and cerebellar lesions.[6,8] This type does not decrease in amplitude or duration with repeated positioning, does not have a clear latency, and usually lasts longer than 30 seconds. The direction is unpredictable and may be different in each position. It is often purely vertical with fast phase directed downward, that is, toward the cheeks.

Gaze-Evoked Nystagmus (Fig. 33)

This type of pathologic nystagmus is induced by having the patient fixate on a target 30 to 40 degrees to the right, left, above, and below the center position. Eye position should be held for at least 30 seconds. Gaze deviation beyond 40 degrees may result in nystagmus even in normal subjects, so-called *end-point nystagmus.* Gaze-evoked nystagmus is prominent with fixation and therefore is readily observed on routine examination.

Patients with *gaze paretic nystagmus* are unable to maintain conjugate eye deviation away from the midposition. Their eyes drift back to the center, requiring corrective fast components toward the periphery. Thus, the nystagmus is

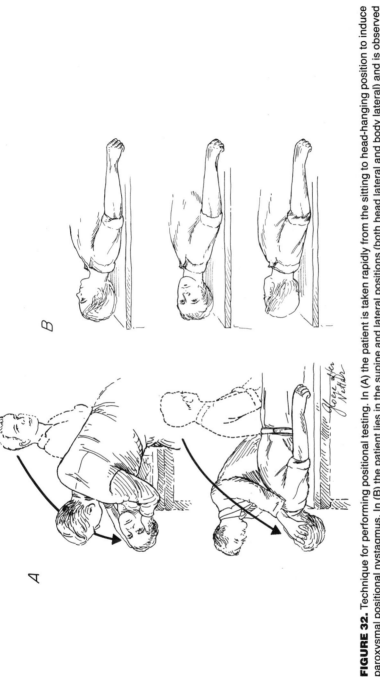

FIGURE 32. Technique for performing positional testing. In (A) the patient is taken rapidly from the sitting to head-hanging position to induce paroxysmal positional nystagmus. In (B) the patient lies in the supine and lateral positions (both head lateral and body lateral) and is observed for static positional nystagmus.

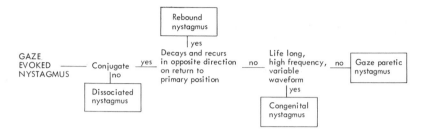

FIGURE 33. Logic for distinguishing between different types of gaze-evoked nystagmus.

always in the direction of gaze and is present with and without fixation. Symmetrical gaze paretic nystagmus is most commonly produced by ingestion of drugs such as phenobarbital, phenytoin, alcohol, and diazepam. It can also occur in patients with such varied conditions as myasthenia gravis, multiple sclerosis, and cerebellar atrophy.[9] Asymmetric horizontal gaze paretic nystagmus always indicates a structural brainstem or cerebellar lesion, with the lesion usually being on the side of the larger amplitude nystagmus (so-called Bruns' nystagmus).

Rebound nystagmus is a type of gaze-evoked nystagmus that either disappears or reverses direction as the eccentric gaze position is held. When the eyes are returned to the primary position, nystagmus occurs in the direction of the return saccade. Thus, the patient may have transient primary position nystagmus in either direction. Rebound nystagmus occurs in patients with cerebellar atrophy and focal structural lesions of the cerebellum; it is the only variety of nystagmus thought to be specific for cerebellar involvement.[10]

The most common variety of *dissociated* (or disconjugate) *nystagmus* results from lesions of the medial longitudinal fasciculus (MLF), so-called internuclear ophthalmoplegia. With horizontal gaze deviation, the adducting eye lags and develops a low amplitude "rounded" nystagmus, while the abducting eye develops a large amplitude nystagmus with a characteristic "sharp peaked" waveform. Patients with myasthenia gravis may develop a similar type of dissociated nystagmus (so-called pseudo-MLF nystagmus), but unlike true MLF nystagmus, the dissociated nystagmus seen with myasthenia progressively increases in amplitude as the gaze position is maintained. Also, unlike MLF nystagmus, pseudo-MLF nystagmus is abolished with edrophonium.

Some varieties of *congenital nystagmus* occur only on lateral gaze, but as with primary position congenital nystagmus, the long history, high frequency, and characteristic waveforms easily distinguish it from other varieties of gaze-evoked nystagmus.

ELECTRONYSTAGMOGRAPHY (ENG)

ENG is a technique for recording eye movements based on the corneal retinal potential (Fig. 34). The pigmented layer of the retina maintains a negative poten-

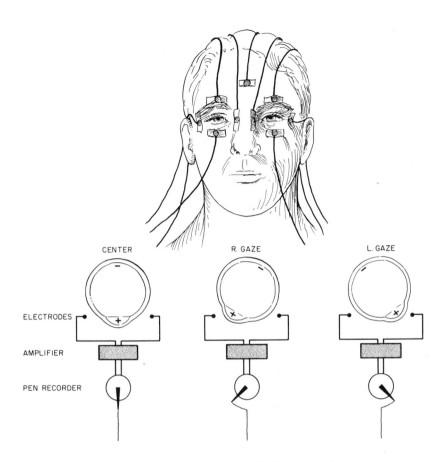

FIGURE 34. Principle of electronystagmography (ENG). See text for details.

tial with regard to the surrounding tissue by means of active ion transport. Because of the sclera's insulating properties the cornea is positive in relation to the retina. Thus, each eye is like a small battery with a surrounding electromagnetic field. In relation to a remote electrode an electrode placed in the vicinity of the eye becomes more positive when the eye rotates towards it, and less positive when it rotates away from it. Recordings are usually made with a three-electrode system using differential amplifiers. Two of the (active) electrodes are placed on each side of the eye and the reference (ground) electrode somewhere remote from the eyes (usually on the forehead). The two active electrodes measure a potential change of equal amplitude, but opposite direction. The difference in potential between these electrodes is amplified and used to control the displacement of a pen-writing recorder or similar device to produce a permanent record. Since the differential amplifiers monitor the difference in voltage between the two active electrodes, remote electric signals (electromyographic or electroencephalographic, for example) arrive at the electrodes with approximately equal amplitude and phase and cancel out.

By convention, for horizontal recordings, eye movements to the right are displayed so that they produce upward pen deflection, and those to the left produce downward deflection (see Fig. 34). For vertical recordings upward and downward, eye movements produce upward and downward deflections respectively. In order to interpret ENG recordings, calibration must be performed so that a standard angle of eye deviation is represented by a known amplitude of pen deflection. Calibration is performed by having the patient maintain his gaze on a series of dots or lights 10 to 20 degrees on each side of, and above and below the central fixation point. Once this relationship is established, the amplitude, duration, and velocity of recorded eye movements can be easily calculated.

With ENG one can quantify the slow component velocity, frequency, and amplitude of pathologic or physiologic nystagmus, and the changes in these measurements brought about by loss of fixation (either with eyes closed or eyes open in darkness). The latter is particularly important, since peripheral vestibular nystagmus often is present only when fixation is inhibited (Fig. 35). As a general rule nystagmus with fixation (nystagmus seen on routine neurologic examination) disappears within one to two weeks after the occurrence of an acute peripheral vestibular lesion. By contrast, peripheral vestibular nystagmus may be recorded with eyes closed for as long as 5 to 10 years after an acute peripheral vestibular lesion.[5] In some patients vestibular nystagmus emerges only when they are mentally alerted (e.g., when performing serial 7 subtractions from 100).

A standard ENG test battery should include tests in 3 major areas: (1) pathologic nystagmus, (2) vestibulo-ocular reflex function, and (3) visual ocular control. Examination for pathologic nystagmus requires a systematic study of (1) changes in fixation (eyes opened fixating, eyes opened in darkness, eyes closed), (2) changes in gaze position (30 degrees left, right, up and down), and (3) changes in head position (supine, head-hanging, and lateral positions). Vestibulo-ocular reflex function is tested with bithermal caloric stimulation and physiologic rotatory stimuli. Examination of visual ocular control includes test of saccades, smooth pursuit, and optokinetic nystagmus (see below).

BITHERMAL CALORIC TESTING

Technique

With bithermal caloric testing each ear is irrigated for a fixed duration (30 to 40 seconds) at a constant flow rate of water that is 7 degrees below body temperature (30°C) and 7 degrees above body temperature (44°C). The patient lies in the supine position with head tilted 30 degrees forward and eyes opened behind Frenzel glasses, or in total darkness. ENG is used to measure the maximum slow phase velocity of each of the four nystagmus responses (Fig. 36). Maximum slow phase velocity is a much more sensitive indicator of vestibular dam-

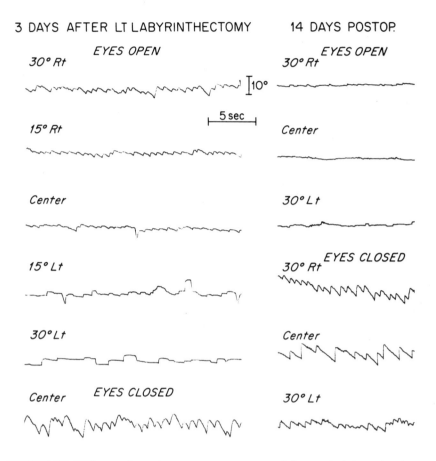

FIGURE 35. ENG recordings of spontaneous nystagmus 3 days and 14 days after the patient underwent a left labyrinthectomy. Nystagmus with eyes opened disappeared by 14 days, but nystagmus with eyes closed remains prominent. (Adapted from Baloh, RW: *Pathologic nystagmus: A classification based on electro-oculographic recordings.* Bull Los Angeles Neurol Soc 41:120, 1976, with permission).

age than the duration of the caloric response.[1] Typically, the average slow phase velocity is calculated for a 5 to 10 second interval at peak response. The major advantages of bithermal caloric testing are: (1) both ampullopetal and ampullofugal endolymph flow are serially induced in each horizontal semicircular canal; (2) the caloric stimulus is reproducible from patient to patient; (3) the magnitude of response is accurately measured; and (4) the test is tolerated by most patients. The major limitation is the need for ENG equipment and constant temperature baths and plumbing to maintain continuous circulation of the water through the infusion hose.

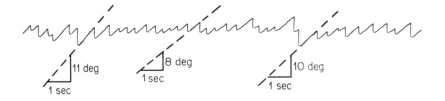

FIGURE 36. ENG recording of caloric-induced nystagmus. The slope of the slow phase gives the slow phase velocity.

The four responses of a bithermal caloric test are routinely compared with two standard formulas (Fig. 37). The vestibular paresis formula

$$\frac{(R30° + R44°) - (L30° + L44°)}{R\,30° + R44° + L30° + L44°} \times 100$$

compares the right-sided responses with the left-sided responses, and the directional preponderance formula

$$\frac{(R30° + L44°) - (R44° + L30°)}{R30° + L44° + R44° + L30°} \times 100$$

compares nystagmus to the right with nystagmus to the left in the same subject. In both of these formulas the difference in response is reported as a percentage of the total response. This is important because the absolute magnitude of caloric response is dependent on several factors, including age.[3] Dividing by the total response normalizes the measurements to remove the large variability in absolute magnitude of normal caloric responses. In our laboratory the upper normal value for vestibular paresis is 22 percent, while that for directional preponderance is 28 percent (using maximum slow phase velocity in the above equations).[4]

A caloric fixation suppression index is obtained by having the patient fixate on a target during the middle of the response. Since the slow phase velocity of caloric-induced nystagmus is constantly changing, it is important that the fixation period occurs near the time of maximum response to obtain the best estimate of fixation suppression. The fixation suppression index is defined as:

$$\frac{\text{Average Slow Phase Velocity With Fixation}}{\text{Average Slow Phase Velocity Without Fixation}} \times 100$$

The average visual suppression index in normal subjects is 48 ± 10 percent.[11]

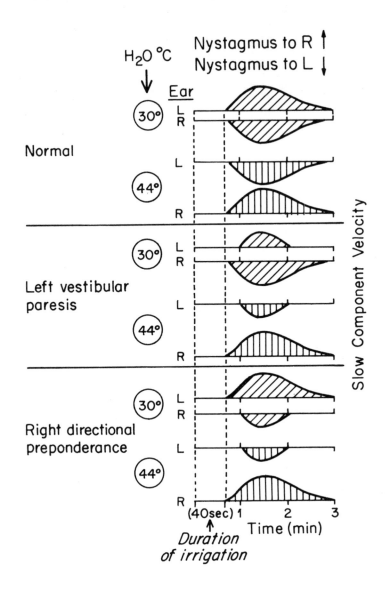

FIGURE 37. Plots of slow component velocity (SCV) vs. time illustrating three characteristic responses to bithermal caloric testing. Normal—peak SCV and duration are symmetrical. Left vestibular paresis—peak SCV and duration are decreased when the left ear is stimulated. Right directional preponderance—peak SCV and duration of nystagmus to the right (L30 and R44) are greater than peak SCV and duration of nystagmus to the left (R30 and L44).

Interpreting Caloric Test Results

As a general rule, a significant *vestibular paresis* on bithermal caloric testing indicates a peripheral vestibular lesion (including the nerve root entry zone), while a significant *directional preponderance* is nonlocalizing (i.e., it can occur with peripheral and central lesions).[1] The latter is often associated with spontaneous nystagmus, in which case the velocity of the slow component of the spontaneous nystagmus adds to that of caloric-induced nystagmus in the same direction and subtracts from that of caloric-induced nystagmus in the opposite direction. The vestibular paresis and directional preponderance formulas are of little use in evaluating patients with bilateral vestibular lesions, since caloric responses are symmetrically depressed. Because of the wide range of normal values for maximum slow phase velocity (5 to 60 deg per sec in our laboratory), the patient's value may decrease several-fold before falling below the normal range. Serial measurements in the same patient are needed if one hopes to identify early bilateral vestibular impairment such as that produced by ototoxic drugs. Also, because of the wide range of normal values it is unusual to find caloric responses that exceed the upper normal range. Lesions of the cerebellum occasionally can lead to bilateral increased caloric responses, apparently owing to the loss of the normal inhibitory influence of the cerebellum on the vestibular nuclei.

Impaired fixation suppression of caloric-induced nystagmus indicates a central nervous system lesion, most commonly a lesion involving the midline cerebellum.[11] Caloric *dysrhythmia* refers to a marked beat-to-beat variability in nystagmus amplitude without any change in the slow component velocity profile.[12] The cerebellum is important for maintaining the regular amplitude of nystagmus fast components, and loss of this control with cerebellar lesions may lead to a disorganized nystagmus pattern (dysrhythmia). *Perverted nystagmus* refers to vertical or oblique nystagmus produced by caloric stimulation of the horizontal semicircular canals.[13] It can occur with many different lesions of the posterior fossa, particularly with lesions in the region of the floor of the fourth ventricle (near the vestibular nuclei). Finally, *disconjugate* caloric-induced nystagmus in which there is a different amplitude and waveform in each eye indicates an intrinsic lesion of the brainstem, most commonly a lesion involving the MLF.

ROTATORY TESTING

Technique

Rotatory tests of the vestibulo-ocular reflexes are not widely used as part of the routine vestibular examination for two reasons: (1) rotatory stimuli affect both labyrinths simultaneously compared with the selective stimulation of one labyrinth possible with caloric tests; and (2) expensive, bulky equipment is required in order to generate precise rotatory stimuli. Rotatory tests do have several advantages, however. Multiple graded stimuli can be applied in a relatively short

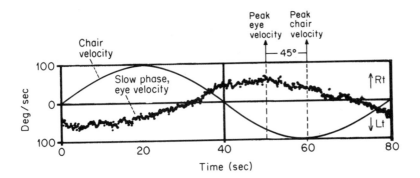

FIGURE 38. Plot of slow phase velocity (SPV) vs. time for nystagmus induced by sinusoidal angular rotation in the horizontal plane (0.0125 Hz, peak velocity—100 deg per sec). Subject is seated on a motorized rotating chair with eyes opened in darkness. Eye movements are recorded with ENG. Fast components are identified and removed and SPV is measured every 20 msec.

period of time, and rotatory testing is usually less bothersome to patients than caloric testing. Unlike caloric testing, a rotatory stimulus to the semicircular canals is unrelated to physical features of the external ear or temporal bone, so that a more exact relationship between stimulus and response is possible.

With rotatory testing, the patient is seated in a chair that rotates about its vertical axis. The head is fixed so that angular rotation occurs in the plane of one of the semicircular canal pairs (usually with the head tilted 30 degrees forward so that rotation occurs in the plane of the horizontal canals). The patient's eyes are opened in complete darkness and the induced nystagmus is recorded with ENG. The gain of the response, defined as the peak slow phase eye velocity divided by the peak chair velocity, is calculated for nystagmus in each direction. In the case of the response illustrated in Figure 38 the gain is 0.6 in both directions.

For sinusoidal rotatory testing, the phase of the response refers to the timing between the maximum velocity of the head and the maximum velocity of the slow phases of nystagmus. This is usually calculated by performing a frequency analysis (Fourier analysis) of the slow phase velocity trace, and comparing the phase of the fundamental frequency to the phase of the head velocity trace. In normal subjects there is a phase lead of eye velocity relative to head velocity at low frequencies (approximately 45 degrees at 0.01 Hz, as illustrated in Fig. 38), but not at higher frequencies (0.2 Hz).

Interpreting Rotatory Test Results

An *asymmetry* in rotatory-induced nystagmus has the same significance as a directional preponderance on bithermal caloric testing; it indicates an imbalance of the vestibulo-ocular reflex, but is nonlocalizing. Patients with a highly significant unilateral vestibular paresis to caloric stimulation may have symmetrical rotatory-induced nystagmus, since the remaining intact labyrinth is able to compensate for the damaged side.[1] For this reason, rotatory testing is not particularly useful for identifying early unilateral peripheral vestibular lesions. An *increase in the low frequency phase lead* of sinusoidal-induced nystagmus is a nonspecific finding that can occur with both peripheral (unilateral and bilateral) and central vestibular lesions.[14] Typically with compensation for a unilateral peripheral vestibular lesion, the asymmetry of rotatory-induced nystagmus disappears within a few months, but the increased phase lead at low frequencies remains for years.[15,16]

Rotatory testing is very useful for evaluating patients with *bilateral peripheral vestibular lesions* (e.g., ototoxic exposure), since both labyrinths are stimulated simultaneously, and the degree of remaining function is accurately quantified. Because the variance associated with normal rotatory responses is less than that associated with caloric responses, diminished function is identified earlier. Artifactually diminished caloric responses occasionally occur in patients with angular, narrow external canals, or with highly pneumatized temporal bones. Since a rotatory stimulus is unrelated to these factors, rotatory-induced nystagmus is normal in such patients. Patients with absent caloric responses may have decreased, but measurable, rotatory-induced nystagmus, particularly at higher stimulus velocities. The ability to identify remaining vestibular function, even if minimal, is an important advantage of rotatory testing, particularly when the physician is contemplating ablative surgery, or monitoring the effects of ototoxic drugs.

Patients with peripheral vestibular lesions, like normal subjects, can suppress physiologic vestibular nystagmus when they are rotated with a fixation point.[14] As with the caloric fixation suppression test, patients with central vestibular lesions (particularly lesions involving the midline cerebellum) often cannot suppress rotatory induced nystagmus with fixation. Rotatory stimuli are ideally suited for evaluating *fixation suppression* of the vestibulo-ocular reflex, since the same precise stimulus can be presented on repeated occasions with and without fixation. Impaired fixation suppression of rotatory-induced nystagmus is nearly always associated with abnormal smooth pursuit.[17] The finding of dysrhythmic, perverted, or disconjugate rotatory-induced nystagmus has the same significance as finding these abnormalities on caloric testing (see prior section).

TESTS OF VISUAL-OCULAR CONTROL

Technique

Along with the vestibulo-ocular reflexes, two visually controlled ocular stabilizing systems produce versional eye movements—the saccadic and smooth pursuit.[18] The saccade system responds to a retinal position error to bring a peripheral target to the fovea in the shortest possible time. The smooth pursuit system maintains gaze on a moving target by generating a continuous match of eye and target velocity. Optokinetic nystagmus is a form of smooth pursuit in which

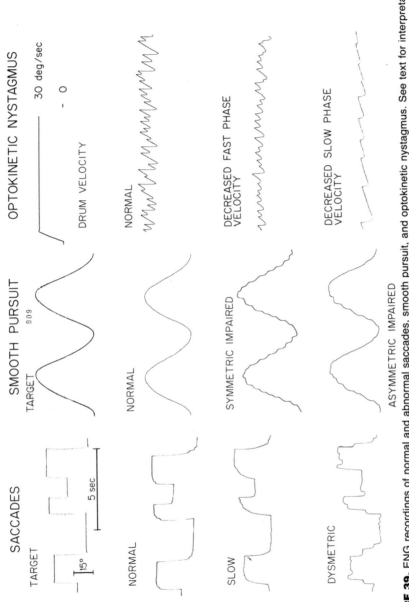

FIGURE 39. ENG recordings of normal and abnormal saccades, smooth pursuit, and optokinetic nystagmus. See text for interpretation of abnormalities.

the eye-tracking motion in one direction is periodically interrupted by corrective saccades in the opposite direction to relocate the gaze on new targets coming into the visual field. Saccadic and pursuit eye movements are induced by having the patient follow a target moving in a step-wise and sinusoidal pattern respectively. For optokinetic testing, a striped pattern is moved across the patient's visual field in a clockwise and counterclockwise direction.

With ENG, features of these visually controlled eye movements can be accurately measured and the results compared with normative data (Fig. 39). One typically measures the peak velocity, accuracy, and reaction time of saccadic eye movements. For pursuit and optokinetic nystagmus, the tracking eye velocity is compared with the target or optokinetic drum velocity.

Interpreting Visual Tracking Test Results

Abnormalities of visual ocular control can be very useful for localizing lesions within the central nervous system (Table 1).[1,19] With one exception, peripheral vestibular lesions do not impair visual ocular control. After an acute unilateral labyrinthine, or vestibular nerve lesion, smooth pursuit and optokinetic slow-phase velocity will be transiently decreased to the contralateral side (i.e., in the direction of the spontaneous nystagmus). The asymmetry in smooth pursuit and optokinetic nystagmus disappears in a few weeks, despite the persistence of vestibular nystagmus in darkness.

Slowing of saccadic eye movements results from lesions anywhere from the horizontal and vertical gaze centers in the paramedian pontine reticular formation and the pretectum, respectively, to the extraocular motor neurons, nerves, and muscles. Lesions involving these structures and interconnecting pathways slow both voluntary saccades and fast components of nystagmus (involuntary saccades) (as illustrated in Fig. 39). Reversible saccade slowing is produced in normal subjects by fatigue and by ingestion of alcohol or tranquilizers. Saccade slowing produced by myasthenia gravis increases with fatigue and is reversed with edrophonium.[20] Lesions of the MLF result in slowing of adducting saccades made by the medial rectus on the side of the lesion.[21] Occasionally, saccade slowing can be identified with ENG recordings when it is not apparent on clinical examination.

Lesions of the supranuclear saccade control centers are often not associated with saccade slowing, but rather with an *alteration in the accuracy or initiation (reaction time) of saccades*. For example, patients with Parkinson's disease exhibit delayed saccade reaction time and hypometric (too small) voluntary saccades.[22] Impaired accuracy is most prominent with cerebellar lesions. Both overshooting and undershooting of the target occur, requiring several corrective saccades to attain the target position *(saccade dysmetria)*. Lesions of the frontal cortex also affect the accuracy of saccades, with saccades to the contralateral side being hypometric. Vertical saccades are unaffected by unilateral cortical lesions.

Patients with impaired smooth pursuit use frequent corrective saccades to keep up with the target, and produce so-called cogwheel or saccadic pursuit (as

TABLE 1. Summary of Visual Ocular Control Abnormalities Produced by Focal Neurologic Lesions[1]

LOCATION OF LESION	SACCADES	SMOOTH PURSUIT	OPTOKINETIC NYSTAGMUS
Unilateral peripheral vestibular	Normal	Transient contralateral impairment	Transient contralateral decreased SCV*
Cerebellopontine angle	Ipsilateral dysmetria†	Progressive ipsilateral or bilateral impairment	Progressive ipsilateral or bilateral decreased SCV
Diffuse cerebellar	Bilateral dysmetria	Bilateral impairment	Bilateral decreased SCV
Intrinsic brain stem	Decreased maximum velocity, increased delay time	Ipsilateral or bilateral impairment	Ipsilateral or bilateral decreased SCV, disconjugate
Basal ganglia	Hypometria,‡ increased delay time (bilateral)	Bilateral impairment	Bilateral decreased SCV
Frontoparietal cortex	Contralateral hypometria	Normal	Normal
Parieto-occipital cortex	Normal	Ipsilateral impairment	Ipsilateral decreased SCV

*slow component velocity
†under and overshoots
‡undershoots only

shown in Fig. 39). The pursuit gain (peak pursuit velocity/peak target velocity) is markedly decreased in such patients. Normal subjects may also intermix saccades with smooth pursuit if the target velocity exceeds the limit of their smooth pursuit system (usually in the range of 60 deg per sec). With ENG, one can use precise stimulus velocities and accurately measure the pursuit velocity between corrective saccades.

Abnormal smooth pursuit occurs with lesions throughout the nervous system.[19] As with saccadic eye movements, tranquilizers, alcohol, and fatigue impair smooth pursuit in normal subjects. Patients with diffuse cortical disease, basal ganglia disease, and cerebellar disease consistently have bilaterally impaired smooth pursuit. Unilateral lesions of the parietal lobe, cerebellum, brain stem, and cerebellopontine angle usually produce ipsilateral impairment of smooth pursuit.[23]

Since optokinetic nystagmus combines pursuit and saccadic eye movements, lesions that affect either or both of these systems produce abnormal optokinetic nystagmus.[24] Symmetrically decreased slow phase velocity occurs with disease of the cortex, diencephalon, brainstem, and cerebellum. As with smooth pursuit, unilateral lesions of the parietal cortex, brainstem, and cerebellum impair optokinetic nystagmus when the stripes move toward the side of the lesion. Patients who cannot generate saccades produce a tonic deviation of the eyes in the direction of the optokinetic stimulus, with absent or small abortive fast components.

COMPUTERIZED ELECTRONYSTAGMOGRAPHY

Digital microcomputers have recently been introduced for on-line analysis of eye movement recordings.[25] With such a system one can obtain quantitative data from patients and make statistical comparisons with normative data within seconds of test completion. The computer controls the stimulus and analyzes the response on-line. The plot of slow phase velocity versus time shown in Fig. 38 is one example of the type of output generated by this system. For these plots, the computer algorithm first identifies and removes fast components (saccades) based on their characteristic velocity profile. By comparing the slow phase eye velocity to the chair velocity during sinusoidal rotatory testing, one can make precise measurements of the vestibulo-ocular reflex gain and phase at different frequencies and peak velocities. Preliminary studies suggest that such measurements are particularly useful for evaluating the response to medical and surgical treatment of vestibular disorders.[15,16]

This same system measures the peak velocity, amplitude, and delay time of voluntary saccades, smooth pursuit velocity after catch-up saccades are removed, and optokinetic slow phase velocity. To date these measurements have proven particularly useful for early detection of multiple sclerosis and myasthenia gravis.[20,26,27]

REFERENCES

1. BALOH, RW, AND HONRUBIA, V: *Clinical Neurophysiology of the Vestibular System.* FA Davis, Philadelphia, 1979.

2. PEITERSEN, E: *Measurement of vestibulo-spinal responses in man.* In KORNHUBER, HH (ED): *Handbook of Sensory Physiology, vol VI, part 2.* Springer-Verlag, New York, 1974.

3. BALOH, RW, SOLINGEN, L, SILLS, A, AND HONRUBIA, V: *Caloric testing. I. Effect of different conditions of ocular fixation.* Ann Otol Rhinol Laryngol, 86(Suppl 43):1, 1977.

4. SILLS, AW, BALOH, RW, AND HONRUBIA, V: *Caloric testing. II. Results in normal subjects.* Ann Otol Rhinol Laryngol 86(Suppl 43):7, 1977.

5. BALOH, RW: *Pathologic nystagmus: A classification based on electro-oculographic recordings.* Bull Los Angeles Neurol Soc 41:120, 1976.

6. HARRISON, MS, AND OZSAHINOGLU, C: *Positional vertigo*. Arch Otolaryngol 101:675, 1975.

7. BALOH, RW, SAKALA, SM, AND HONRUBIA, V: *Benign paroxysmal positional nystagmus*. Am J Otolaryngol 1:1, 1979.

8. HALLPIKE, CS: *Vertigo of central origin*. Proc Roy Soc Med 55:364, 1962.

9. COGAN, DG: *Neurology of the Ocular Muscles*. Charles C Thomas, Springfield, Illinois, 1956.

10. HOOD, JD, KAYAN, A, AND LEECH, J: *Rebound nystagmus*. Brain 96:507, 1973.

11. TAKEMORI, S, AND COHEN, B: *Loss of visual suppression of vestibular nystagmus after flocculus lesions*. Brain Res 72:213, 1974.

12. RIESCO-MCCLURE, J, AND STROUD, M: *Dysrhythmia in the post-caloric nystagmus. Its clinical significance*. Laryngoscope 70:697, 1960.

13. FREDRICKSON, JM, AND FERNANDEZ, C: *Vestibular disorders in fourth ventricle lesions*. Arch Otolaryngol 80:521, 1964.

14. BALOH, RW, YEE, RD, JENKINS, HA, AND HONRUBIA, V: *Quantitative assessment of visual-vestibular interaction using sinusoidal rotatory stimuli*. In HONRUBIA, V AND BRAZIER, AB (EDS): *Nystagmus and Vertigo*. Academic Press, New York, 1982.

15. WOLFE, JW, ENGELKEN, EJ, AND OLSON, JE: *Low-frequency harmonic acceleration in the evaluation of patients with peripheral labyrinthine disorders*. In HONRUBIA, V, AND BRAZIER, AB (EDS): *Nystagmus and Vertigo*. Academic Press, New York, 1982.

16. HONRUBIA, V, JENKINS, HA, BALOH, RW, AND LAU, CGY: *Evaluation of rotatory tests in peripheral labyrinthine lesions*. In HONRUBIA, V, AND BRAZIER, AB (EDS): *Nystagmus and Vertigo*. Academic Press, New York, 1982.

17. DICHGANS, J, VON REUTERN, GM, AND ROMMELT V: *Impaired suppression of vestibular nystagmus by fixation in cerebellar and noncerebellar patients*. Arch Psychiatr Nervenkr 226:183, 1978.

18. LEIGH, J, AND ZEE, D: *The Neurology of Eye Movements. (Contemporary Neurology Series)*. FA Davis, Philadelphia, 1983.

19. BALOH, RW, HONRUBIA, V, AND SILLS, A: *Eye-tracking and optokinetic nystagmus. Results of quantitative testing in patients with well-defined nervous system lesions*. Ann Otol Rhinol Laryngol 86:108, 1977.

20. BALOH, RW, AND KEESEY, JC: *Saccade fatigue and response to edrophonium for the diagnosis of myasthenia gravis*. Ann NY Acad Sci 274:631, 1976.

21. BALOH, RW, YEE, RD, AND HONRUBIA, V: *Internuclear ophthalmoplegia. I. Saccades and dissociated nystagmus*. Arch Neurol 35:484, 1978.

22. DEJONG, JD, AND MELVILL-JONES, G: *Akinesia, hypokinesia and bradykinesia in the oculomotor system of patients with Parkinson's disease*. Exp Neurol 32:58, 1971.

23. BALOH, RW, YEE, RD, AND HONRUBIA, V: *Optokinetic nystagmus and parietal lobe lesions*. Ann Neurol 7:269, 1980.

24. BALOH, RW, YEE, RD, AND HONRUBIA, V: *Clinical abnormalities of optokinetic nystagmus.* In LENNERSTRAND, G, ZEE, DS, AND KELLER, EL (EDS): *Functional Basis of Ocular Motility Disorders.* Pergamon Press, New York, 1982.

25. BALOH, RW, LANGHOFER, L, HONRUBIA, V, AND YEE, RD: *On-line analysis of eye movements using a digital computer.* Aviat Space Environ Med 51:563, 1980.

26. SOLINGEN, LD, BALOH, RW, MYERS, L, AND ELLISON, G: *Subclinical eye movement disorders in patients with multiple sclerosis.* Neurology 27:614, 1977.

27. MASTAGLIA, FL, BLACK, JL, AND COLLINS, DWK: *Quantitative studies of saccadic and pursuit eye movements in multiple sclerosis.* Brain 102:817, 1979.

8

EXAMINATION OF THE AUDITORY SYSTEM

BEDSIDE TESTS

A quick test for hearing loss in the speech range is to observe the response to spoken commands at different intensities (whisper, conversation, shouting). The examiner stands behind the patient to prevent lip reading, and occludes and masks the non-test ear by moving a finger back and forth in the patient's external ear canal. A high frequency stimulus such as a watch tick or coin click (approximately 4,000 cps) can also be used, since sensorineural disorders often involve only the higher frequencies. Tuning fork tests permit a rough assessment of the hearing level for pure tones of known frequency. The clinician can use his own hearing level as a reference standard. The *Rinne test* compares the patient's hearing by air conduction with that by bone conduction. The fork (preferably 512 cps) is first held against the mastoid process until the sound fades. It is then placed one inch from the ear. Normal subjects can hear the fork about twice as long by air as by bone conduction. If bone conduction is greater than air conduction, a conductive hearing loss is suggested. The *Weber test* compares the patient's hearing by bone conduction in the two ears. The fork is placed at the center of the forehead or on a central incisor, and the patient is asked where he hears the tone. Normal subjects hear it in the center of the head, patients with unilateral conductive loss hear it on the affected side, and patients with unilateral sensorineural loss hear it on the side opposite the loss.

STANDARD AUDIOMETRY

Audiometry typically consists of a battery of tests, the differential results of which provide site-of-lesion information.[1]

Pure Tone Studies

Pure tones are defined by their frequency and intensity. In order to quantify the magnitude of hearing loss, normal hearing levels for pure tones are defined by an international standard. These levels approximate the intensity of the faintest sound that can be heard by normal ears. A patient's hearing level is the difference in decibels (dB) between the faintest pure tone that he can hear and the normal reference level given by the standard. Brief duration pure tones at selected frequencies are presented via earphones (air conduction) and a vibrator pressed against the mastoid portion of the temporal bone (bone conduction). The results of air and bone conduction testing are plotted on an audiogram from which the magnitude (in dB) and configuration (sensitivity loss as a function of frequency) of the hearing loss can be determined (Fig. 40).

With conductive hearing loss, air conduction is impaired, while bone conduction remains normal (i.e., an air-bone gap on the audiogram, see Fig. 40). Measurement of bone conduction requires careful masking of the non-test ear, since a failure to use masking may result in a false impression of inner ear function. Masking involves introducing a noise into the non-test ear to eliminate inaccurate threshold levels that result from cross-hearing. There is less than a 5 dB attenuation between the two ears for a bone conduction receiver placed on any part of the skull.[2] Therefore, a non-hearing ear may appear to have near-normal hearing via bone conduction if the normal ear is not properly masked. The best masking sound for pure tones is a narrow band of white noise centered about the pure tone being tested.

Lesions producing sensorineural hearing loss impair both air and bone conduction, often with changing pure tone levels at different frequencies. Typical audiogram pure tone patterns seen in patients with four common causes of sensorineural hearing loss are shown in Figure 41. None of these patterns is pathognomonic of a given disorder but they occur often enough to be of diagnostic use.

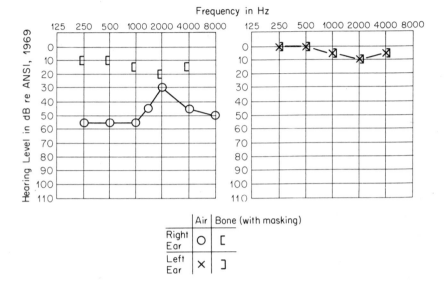

FIGURE 40. Pure tone audiogram: left ear—normal; right ear—conductive hearing loss due to otosclerosis.

Speech Studies

Two types of tests are used to determine the patient's ability to hear and understand speech. The *speech reception threshold* (SRT) is the intensity at which the patient can correctly repeat 50 percent of highly familiar two-syllable words (e.g., airplane, cowboy, sidewalk, etc.). The SRT is an estimate of the minimum level of conversation which a person can hear. It provides a check on the validity of the pure-tone tests, since it should agree with an average of the two best pure-tone thresholds on the audiogram (± 5 dB). It is not a test of discrimination, but it does provide information about a patient's ability to recognize and respond to speech.

The *speech discrimination* test is a measure of the patient's ability to understand speech when it is presented at a level that is easily heard. For this test the patient is usually presented with 50 phonetically balanced monosyllabic words at a comfortable listening level. Each word is presented with a carrier phrase such as "You will say ____" or "Say the word ____." The test is scored as a percentage of the correct responses, e.g., 49 out of 50 correct = 98 percent speech discrimination. In patients with VIII nerve lesions, speech discrimination can be severely reduced even when pure tone thresholds are normal or near normal, whereas in patients with cochlear lesions discrimination tends to be proportional to the magnitude of hearing loss.[3]

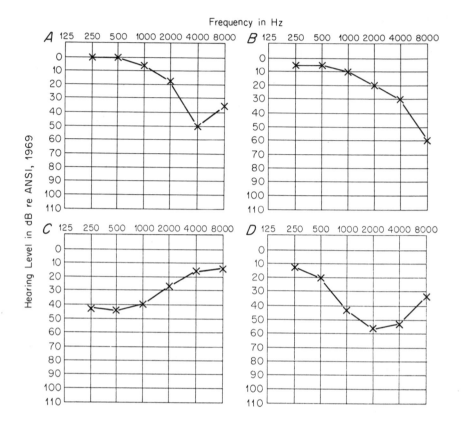

FIGURE 41. Audiograms illustrating four characteristic patterns of sensorineural hearing loss. (A) Notched pattern of noise induced hearing loss; (B) downward sloping pattern of presbycusis; (C) low frequency trough of Meniere's syndrome; and (D) V-pattern of congenital hearing loss.

Recruitment

The alternate binaural loudness balance (ABLB) test provides a direct measurement of loudness recruitment if the hearing loss is unilateral. A short duration tone is presented alternately to each ear. The intensity of the tone to one ear is fixed, while the intensity to the other ear is adjusted until the listener perceives the loudness of the two tones to be equal. Recruitment of loudness is present if the patient requires a smaller intensity increase (above threshold in quiet) in the hearing impaired ear than is required in the better hearing ear to achieve equal loudness between the two ears. Recruitment is typically seen with lesions involving the cochlea.

Tone Decay

Tone decay can be measured using a continuously variable or automatic (Bekesy-type) audiometer.[4] In either case, a stimulus is presented continuously at the starting intensity level and the examiner records the length of time the stimulus is audible to the patient. Under the manual presentation method the examiner increases the intensity of the signal until the patient can perceive the tone for 60 seconds at a constant intensity level. Using the Bekesy audiometer, a graphic representation of the intensity level required for the patient to maintain audibility of the tone is obtained. Abnormal tone decay is typically seen with lesions involving the auditory nerve.

IMPEDANCE AUDIOMETRY

Impedance may be defined as the resistance of a given system to the flow of energy. Acoustic impedance refers to the resistance of the middle ear system to the passage of sound. Its reciprocal, acoustic compliance, refers to the ease of sound transmission through the middle ear system. In simplified terms, acoustic impedance indicates the stiffness of the middle ear conduction system, while acoustic compliance describes the mobility or springiness of the same system. Measurement of acoustic impedance is based on the principle that sound pressure level (SPL) varies with the volume of a closed cavity such as the external ear canal.[5] For a given tone of known frequency and intensity, the SPL decreases as cavity size increases. By measuring the difference between the intensity of a sound going into the external auditory canal and that reflected back from the tympanic membrane, one can estimate the stiffness (or compliance) of the middle ear system.

Acoustic impedance measurements are made via a probe tip hermetically inserted into the ear canal. The probe tip contains three openings: (1) one for air pressure generation and measurement; (2) one for probe tone generation; and (3) one for pickup of sound waves reflected off the tympanic membrane. A schematic drawing of the impedance measurement system is shown in Figure 42. With this system, the difference between generated and reflected sound is systematically measured at different external ear pressure levels.

Static Measurements

A normal middle ear and tympanic membrane offer relatively low acoustic impedance, implying that appreciable energy is absorbed and transmitted through the middle ear. If the middle ear contains fluid, or the tympanic membrane is sclerotic, the acoustic impedance is increased and the transmission capability is diminished, that is, the static compliance is decreased. An increase in acoustic impedance can also result from a decrease in flexibility of the ossicular chain, an increase in its mass, or an increase in friction during ossicular movement. An ossicular chain discontinuity causes a decrease in acoustic impedance, since the mass and friction decrease. Unfortunately, acoustic impe-

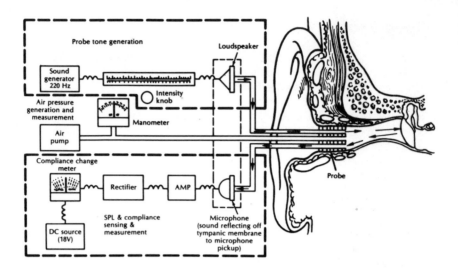

FIGURE 42. Schematic drawing of acoustic impedance measuring system. See text for details. (From Goodhill, V: *Ear Diseases, Deafness and Dizziness.* Harper and Row, Hagerstown, MD, 1979, with permission).

dance and static compliance measurements rarely provide critical diagnostic information, since the range of normal values is large, and there is overlap in values for different otologic disorders.

Tympanometry

Tympanometry is a method for evaluating changes in acoustic impedance by producing systematic changes in air pressure in the external ear canal. A plot of compliance change versus air pressure (tympanogram) is made by first introducing a positive pressure into the external canal (usually equivalent to $+200$ mm H_2O), and then decreasing the pressure to approximately -200 mm H_2O (although the negative range can be extended to -600 mm H_2O). As the pressure is changed, compliance will change if the conduction system is normal. The shape of a normal tympanogram resembles a tepee (Fig. 43). The peak of the tepee represents the point of maximum compliance where the air pressure in the middle ear equals the air pressure in the external auditory canal. Tympanometry can provide useful information about (1) mobility of the tympanic membrane, (2) perforations of the tympanic membrane, (3) pressure within the middle ear, and (4) patency and dynamic function of the eustachian tubes.

Four characteristic abnormal tympanographic patterns can be identified (see Fig. 43).[6,7] A restricted tympanogram implies normal middle ear pressure and limited compliance relative to normal mobility. It is typically seen in advanced cases of otosclerosis, lateral fixation of the ossicular chain, tympanic

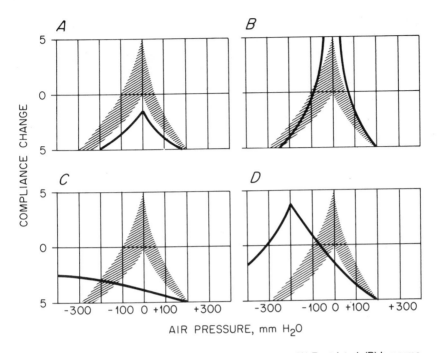

FIGURE 43. Four characteristic abnormal tympanograms. (A) Restricted, (B) hypermobile, (C) flat, and (D) retracted. Striped area—normal range.

membrane fibrosis, and middle ear tympanosclerosis. A hypermobile tympanogram indicates a flaccid tympanic membrane. It occurs with ossicular chain discontinuity and with partial atrophy of the tympanic membrane. A flat tympanogram means that there is little or no change in middle ear compliance when air pressure is varied in the external ear canal. This pattern is most commonly seen with serous otitis media, but can also be seen with congenital malformations of the middle ear and occlusion of the external ear canal by cerumen, epithelium, and foreign bodies. Finally, with a retracted tympanogram the maximum compliance occurs at negative pressures greater than –100 mm H_2O. It implies a negative middle ear pressure with a retracted tympanic membrane. This pattern is most commonly seen with poor eustachian tube function.

The Acoustic Reflex

The acoustic reflex refers to contraction of the stapedius muscle in response to a loud sound (see Fig. 22). It is measured by monitoring the change in acoustic impedance in response to a loud sound introduced into either ear. The stapedius muscle contracts bilaterally, regardless of which ear is stimulated. Contraction of the stapedius muscle produces stiffening of the tympanic membrane, and thus an increase in acoustic impedance. This results in an attenuation of sound transmitted to the cochlea by about 10 dB. In a normal subject the acoustic reflex will be observed when a pure tone signal is presented between 70-100 dB above hearing level (median value 82 dB), and when a white noise stimulus is presented at 65 dB above hearing level.[8]

The stimulus sound can be presented to either the contralateral ear, or to the ear with the recording probe tip. In the former case one tests the contralateral VIII nerve, brainstem crossover pathways, and the ipsilateral VII nerve and middle ear system. In the latter case one tests the ipsilateral VIII nerve, ipsilateral brainstem connections, and the ipsilateral VII nerve and middle ear system. By systematically presenting the stimulus sound to each ear and recording with the probe tip in each ear, the location of a lesion within the reflex pathway can be isolated. The results of acoustic reflex testing in patients with four different common unilateral lesions are summarized in Table 2.

Patients with conductive hearing loss often have an absent reflex because the lesion prevents a change in compliance with stapedius muscle contraction. An air-bone gap as small as 5 dB may obscure the acoustic reflex.[9] The acoustic reflex is particularly useful for identifying the site of lesion for different types of sensorineural hearing loss. With cochlear lesions, the acoustic reflex often can be demonstrated at a sensation level less than 60 dB above the auditory pure-tone threshold. This is another form of abnormal loudness growth or recruitment. A cochlear hearing loss must be severe before the acoustic reflex is lost. An absent reflex is rarely associated with a cochlear hearing loss less than 50 dB, and only when the hearing loss exceeds 85 dB is the reflex absent in 50 percent of patients.[10] By contrast, patients with VIII nerve lesions often have either normal hearing, or only mildly impaired hearing (less than 20 dB), yet have an abnormal acoustic reflex. The reflex may be absent, exhibit an elevated threshold, or exhibit abnormal decay. Reflex decay is present if the amplitude decreases to one-half of its original size within 10 seconds of tonal stimulation. The acoustic reflex is abnormal in approximately 80 percent of patients with surgically documented acoustic neuromas.[11]

TABLE 2. Pattern of acoustic reflex measurements with unilateral lesions

	*C	I	C	I
STIMULUS PRESENTED: REFLEX MEASURED:	†I	C	C	I
Type of Lesion				
Cochlear (<85dB HL)	+	+	+	+
Conductive (>30dB HL)	−	−	+	−
VIII nerve	+	−	+	−
VII nerve	−	+	+	−

*Contralateral to lesion
†Ipsilateral to lesion
Plus sign—reflex present
Minus sign—reflex absent

AUDITORY EVOKED RESPONSES

The advent of averaging computers has made it possible to collect and analyze a variety of evoked electrical potentials from the auditory nervous system.[12] Disk electrodes are attached to the head, repetitive sounds are delivered to the external ear, and an "averaged" series of specific brain wave potentials for up to 500 msec after signal onset can be recorded. The latencies (re: signal onset) of each of the brain wave potentials are used as the most reliable means by which generator sources for the potentials in the central nervous system are identified. Specifically, the early (0 to 10 msec) evoked responses reflect the far field representation of electrical events generated at points from the periphery (VIII nerve action potential) to the level of the brainstem. The five to seven waves in the first 10 msec are referred to as the brainstem evoked response. The middle latency responses (12 to 50 msec) have received less systematic study, but probably reflect electrical activity in the upper brainstem and in the primary and nearby secondary auditory projection areas. The late evoked responses (50 to 300 msec) reflect cortical electrical activity.

The brainstem auditory evoked response (BAER) is highly reproducible in a given subject, and shows little variation among normal subjects. With rare exceptions, the BAER is not affected by inattention to the stimulus, alterations in the level of consciousness, or drugs. For this reason it can be used to test the integrity of the peripheral and brainstem auditory pathways in patients who cannot cooperate with subjective auditory testing (e.g., infants, comatose patients, etc.).

A schematic drawing of a BAER and the neuronal centers that are thought to generate each component of the response is shown in Figure 44. Wave I (average latency 1.9 msec) results from activation of the VIII nerve terminals within the cochlea, while the remainder of the waves are generated by the retrocochlear part of the VIII nerve and the brainstem auditory nuclei and pathways.[13,14,15] Although a useful working tool, this schematic electroanatomic correlation is an oversimplification. Clearly each vertex-positive and vertex-negative potential after wave I reflects simultaneous activity in multiple brainstem loci. The more caudal generators, such as the VIII nerve, cochlear nuclei, and superior olivary complex contribute to the response beyond waves II and III. By the time waves VI and VII appear, the summation of potentials from the different neuronal centers is so complex that the concept of single principal contributors to individual waves no longer applies. Therefore, the greatest diagnostic value of BAER is to establish the presence of a central lesion, rather than to define its precise location.

The standard stimulus for eliciting BAERs is a click caused by a very short DC pulse. This is a spectrally diffused acoustic stimulus with most of the energy concentrated in the high frequencies (2000 Hz). The absolute latency of the BAER waves is dependent on the intensity of the click stimulus. The BAERs to unfiltered clicks presented at various intensity levels from a normal subject are shown in Figure 45. Wave V is most robust, often being identifiable at only 10 dB above hearing level. At 60 dB above hearing level, all waves are identifiable.

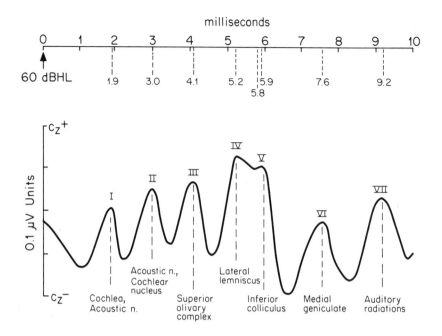

FIGURE 44. Normal brainstem auditory response evoked by clicks of 60 dB HL (60 dB above normal hearing threshold) at a rate of 10 per second. Normal mean latencies for waves I through VII are shown on the time scale (the intermediate latency, 5.8 ms, between waves IV and V is the mean peak latency of a fused wave IV/V when present). The neural centers thought to be responsible for generating each wave are shown at the bottom. (Adapted from Stockard, JJ, Stockard, JE and Sharbrough, FW: *Detection and localization of occult lesions with brain stem auditory responses.* Mayo Clinic Proc 52:761, 1977.)

Such latency-intensity functions provide a basis for estimating the degree of hearing loss in patients who cannot cooperate with standard pure-tone testing.[16,17] On the other hand, because of this latency-intensity relationship, BAERs must be interpreted with caution in patients with severe conductive or cochlear hearing loss (particularly if it involves the high frequencies).

In practice, only waves I, III, and V are used to define response abnormalities. Waves II, IV, VI, and VII are sufficiently variable in the normal population to preclude their routine use in defining response abnormalities on the basis of a single recording. Often waves IV and V fuse into a single complex, which is designated as wave IV/V. Since wave I disappears before wave IV/V with decreasing stimulus intensity (e.g., see Fig. 45), the absence of wave IV/V in the presence of wave I indicates a lesion of the VIII nerve. The absence of all waves, on the other hand, often reflects a peripheral lesion (conductive or cochlear), or

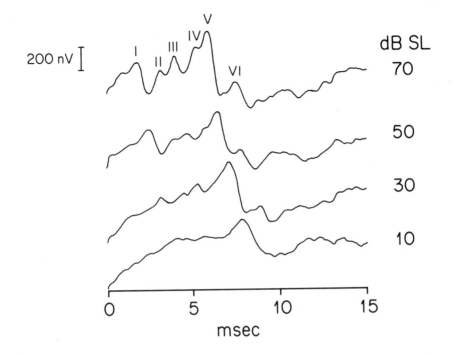

FIGURE 45. Brainstem auditory evoked responses in a normal subject induced by clicks at varying intensity levels (10 to 70 dB SL, sensation level).

a technical problem.[14,18] If peak I occurs at normal latency then prolongation of the I–III or I–IV/V interval indicates a lesion of the VIII nerve or brainstem.

BAER measurements have been particularly useful for early detection of acoustic neuromas. Abnormal BAERs occur in approximately 95 percent of surgically proven cases.[19,20] The most common abnormality overall is absence of all waves beyond wave I. For small tumors with minimal or no detectable pure tone hearing loss, prolongation of the I–IV/V interval is the most common finding (Fig. 46).

CENTRAL AUDITORY SPEECH TESTS

Patients with lesions of the central auditory pathways usually have pure tone thresholds within the normal range. Routine speech tests are also usually normal, since speech contains a great deal of redundancy. Within the central auditory pathways redundancy is enhanced by the multiple crossings and interactions. One of the few diagnostically useful clinical audiologic findings is the reduced ability of patients with temporal lobe lesions to discriminate speech in the ear contralateral to the lesion when the task is complicated by distorting the

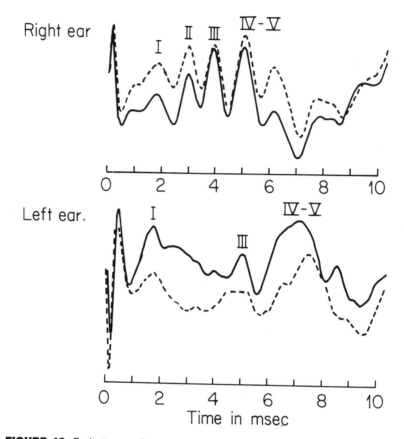

FIGURE 46. Brainstem auditory evoked responses in a patient with a left acoustic neuroma. Dashed lines indicate repeat test. Wave I occurs at normal latency on both sides but the I–III and I–V interval are prolonged on the left side. (Courtesy D Morgan, Ph.D., Audiology, UCLA).

speech.[21] Apparently by making the speech less redundant, heavier demands are placed on the integrating and synthesizing function of the auditory cortex.

There are several varieties of central auditory speech tests currently in use, each involving different methods of presenting distorted speech.[1,21] Portions of the frequency spectrum of speech can be filtered, the speech can be time compressed, it can be presented at very low intensities, and the speech can be interrupted at irregular intervals. Dichotic stimulation involves presenting two different messages to each ear. Both monosyllabic and spondee words can be used. As with distorted speech tests when a temporal lobe lesion exists, the ear contralateral to the lesion performs poorer than the ear ipsilateral to the lesion.

REFERENCES

1. KATZ, J (ED): *Handbook of Clinical Audiology,* ED 2. Williams and Wilkins, Baltimore, 1977.

2. HEFFERNAN, HP, SIMONS, MR, AND GOODHILL, V: *Audiologic assessment, functional hearing loss and objective audiometry.* In GOODHILL, V (ED): *Ear Diseases, Deafness and Dizziness.* Harper and Row, Hagerstown, Maryland, 1979.

3. JERGER, J, AND JERGER, S: *Diagnostic significance of PB word functions.* Arch Otolaryngol 93:573, 1971.

4. HEFFERNAN, HP, AND SIMONS, MR: *Conductive loss and sensorineural test batteries.* In GOODHILL, V (ED): *Ear Diseases, Deafness and Dizziness.* Harper and Row, Hagerstown, Maryland, 1979.

5. SIMONS, MR: *Acoustic impedance tests.* In GOODHILL, V (ED): *Ear Diseases, Deafness and Dizziness.* Harper and Row, Hagerstown, Maryland, 1979.

6. LIDEN, G, PEDERSON, JL, BJORKMAN, G: *Tympanometry.* Arch Otolaryngol 92:248, 1970.

7. JERGER, J: *Clinical experience with impedance audiometry.* Arch Otolaryngol 92:311, 1970.

8. JEPSON, O: *Middle ear muscle reflexes in man.* In JERGER, J (ED): *Modern Developments in Audiology.* Academic Press, New York, 1963.

9. JERGER, J, ANTHONY, L, JERGER, S, et al: *Studies in impedance audiometry. III. Middle ear disorders.* Arch Otolaryngol 99:165, 1974.

10. JERGER, J, JERGER, S, AND MAULDEN, L: *Studies in impedance audiometry. I. Normal and S-N ears.* Arch Otolaryngol 96:513, 1972.

11. SHEEHY, JL, AND INZER, BE: *Acoustic reflex test in neurotologic diagnosis.* Arch Otolaryngol 102:647, 1976.

12. GALAMBOS, R: *Electrophysiological measurement of human auditory function.* In EAGLES, EL (ED): *Human Communication and Its Disorders, vol 3.* Raven Press, New York, 1975.

13. STARR, A, AND HAMILTON, AE: *Correlation between confirmed sites of neurological lesions and abnormalities of far-field auditory brainstem responses.* Electroencephalogr Clin Neurophysiol 41:595, 1976.

14. STOCKARD, JJ, STOCKARD, JE, AND SHARBROUGH, FW: *Detection and localization of occult lesions with brainstem auditory responses.* Mayo Clinic Proc 52:761, 1977.

15. MØLLER, AR, JANETTA, PJ, MØLLER, MB: *Neural generators of brainstem evoked potentials. Results from human intracranial recordings.* Ann Otol Rhinol Laryngol 90:591, 1981.

16. DON, M, EGGERMONT, JJ, AND BRACHMANN, DE: *Reconstruction of the audiogram using brain stem responses and high-pass noise masking.* Ann Otol Rhinol Laryngol 88 (Suppl 57):1, 1979.

17. DAVIS, H: *Auditory evoked potentials as a method for assessing hearing impairment.* Trends in NeuroSciences p 126, June, 1981.

18. COATS, AC: *Human auditory nerve action potentials and brain stem evoked responses.* Arch Otolaryngol 104:799, 1978.

19. CLEMIS, JD, MCGEE, T: *Brain stem electric response audiometry in the differential diagnosis of acoustic tumors.* Laryngoscope 89:31, 1979.

20. JOSEY, AF, JACKSON, GG, GLASSCOCK, ME: *Brainstem evoked response audiometry in confirmed eighth nerve tumors.* Am J Otolaryngol 1:285, 1980.

21. BERLIN, C, LOWE-BELL, S, JANETTA, P AND KLINE, D: *Central auditory deficits after temporal lobectomy.* Arch Otolaryngol 96:4, 1972.

PART 3
DIAGNOSIS AND TREATMENT

9

CAUSES OF NEUROTOLOGIC SYMPTOMS

INFECTION
  Acute Otitis Media
  Chronic Otomastoiditis
  Bacterial Labyrinthitis
  Intracranial Complications of Otitic Infections
  Viral Labyrinths
  Viral Neuritis
  Syphilitic Infections

VASCULAR DISORDERS
  Vertebrobasilar Insufficiency
  Migraine
  Benign Paroxysmal Vertigo of Childhood
  Labyrinthine Infarction
  Cogan's Syndrome
  Brainstem Infarction
  Cerebellar Infarction
  Intralabyrinthine Hemorrhage
  Cerebellar Hemorrhage
  Brainstem Hemorrhage

MENIERE'S SYNDROME (ENDOLYMPHATIC HYDROPS)

DEGENERATIVE DISORDERS OF THE LABYRINTH
  Benign Paroxysmal Positional Vertigo
  Effects of Aging on the Auditory
    and Vestibular Systems

TUMORS
  Primary Carcinoma
  Metastatic Carcinoma
  Glomus Body Tumors
  Acoustic Neuroma
  Other Cerebellopontine Angle Tumors

DEVELOPMENTAL DISORDERS
  Congenital Malformations of the Inner Ear
  Malformations of the Craniovertebral Junction

TRAUMA
  Temporal Bone Fracture
  Labyrinthine Concussion
  Perilymph Fistula
  Otitic Barotrauma
  Noise-Induced Hearing Loss
  Surgery

OTOSCLEROSIS

PAGET'S DISEASE

DIABETES MELLITUS

TOXINS
  Aminoglycosides
  Salicylates
  Other Ototoxic Drugs
  Alcohol

BELL'S PALSY

MULTIPLE SCLEROSIS

CERVICAL VERTIGO

INFECTION

Acute Otitis Media

Acute inflammation of the middle ear (acute otitis media) is a common cause of conductive hearing loss, particularly in children.[1] Either infected (suppurative otitis) or noninfected (serous otitis) fluid accumulates in the middle ear, impairing conduction of airborne sound. Since the air cavity of the middle ear is in direct connection with the mastoid air cells, infection can spread throughout the pneumatized parts of the temporal bone (see Fig. 1). The flow chart in Figure 47 summarizes typical patterns of progression of middle ear infections.

Inflammation of the middle ear probably accompanies every viral upper respiratory tract infection (URI). The nasal, paranasal, and pharyngeal muco-

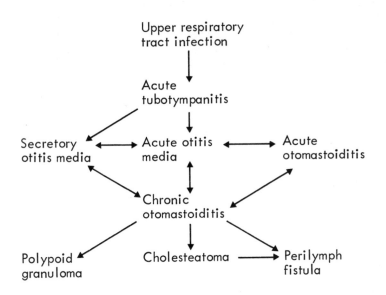

FIGURE 47. Typical patterns of progression of middle ear infections.

sitis spreads to involve the eustachian tube and middle ear mucosa, producing a *tubotympanitis.* As noted in Chapter 1, the mucosa of the pharyngeal end of the eustachian tube is continuous with the mucociliary system of the middle ear. Tubotympanitis accompanying most URIs is transitory, and subsides without significant sequela. In a small percentage of cases, however, a secondary bacterial superinfection occurs, producing acute bacterial otitis media.[2] Common etiologic organisms are Haemophilus influenzae in infants and young children, and Streptococcus pneumoniae in older children and adults. Acute otitis media commonly progresses to spontaneous tympanic membrane rupture and otorrhea. Persistent acute otitis media can lead to secretory otitis media or to acute otomastoiditis. The most direct route for infection to spread into the mastoid is through the aditus ad antrum.

Chronic Otomastoiditis

Chronic otomastoiditis results from untreated or nonresponsive acute otomastoiditis, or secretory otitis media. In addition to the conductive hearing loss common with acute infection, ears with chronic infection have an increased incidence of sensorineural hearing loss.[3,4] The pathology of chronic otomastoiditis is characterized by thickened edematous mucosa, with obliteration of the mastoid air cell lumens, perivascular fibrosis, and osteitis.[5] *Polypoid granulomas* composed of hyperplastic mucosa may fill the mastoid antrum, extend into the middle ear, and extrude through a tympanic membrane perforation into the external auditory canal. *Keratinizing squamous epithelium (cholesteatoma)* can in-

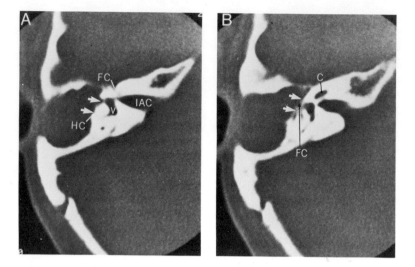

FIGURE 48. CT scan of the temporal bone in a patient with a cholesteatoma eroding the wall of the horizontal semicircular canal (A) and the facial canal (B). Arrows point toward area of bony erosion: FC—facial canal, HSC—horizontal semicircular canal, V—vestibule, IAC—internal auditory canal (Courtesy William Hanafee, M.D. and Sven Larsen, M.D., Radiology, UCLA).

vade the middle ear and other pneumatized areas of the temporal bone through a chronic perforation in the tympanic membrane. Cholesteatomas usually develop in the epitympanic space after penetrating a perforation in the pars flaccida region of the tympanic membrane (see Fig. 3B). From here they extend posteriorly into the antrum, into the central mastoid tract or inferiorly into the middle ear to erode the ossicles and bony labyrinth, producing a mixed conductive-sensorineural hearing loss and vertigo (Fig. 48). A cholesteatoma may accumulate slowly for years or may develop rapidly with a recurrent infection. When infected, the cholesteatoma may erode through the temporal bone into the intracranial cavity, producing central nervous system symptoms and signs.

Also, with chronic otomastoiditis a *fistula* may develop in the bony labyrinth, producing an artificial communication between perilymph and the middle ear. The fistula is caused by either progressive rarefying osteitis or erosion by a cholesteatoma (see Fig. 48). Patients with a perilymph fistula experience incapacitating episodes of vertigo when they sneeze or cough because the sudden change in middle ear pressure is transmitted directly to the inner ear. A perilymph fistula can be identified on examination by transiently changing the pressure in the external canal, using a pneumatic bulb attached to an otoscope. With a positive fistula test the patient develops vertigo and nystagmus lasting 10 to 20 seconds.

Bacterial Labyrinthitis

Invasion of the labyrinth by bacteria is an infrequent occurrence since the introduction of antibiotics. With otitis media, bacteria can enter the inner ear through the oval or round windows, or by eroding through the bony walls. Patients with bacterial meningitis may develop labyrinthitis when bacteria enter the perilymphatic space from the cerebrospinal fluid via the cochlear aqueduct or internal auditory canal (Fig. 49). Bacterial labyrinthitis invariably leads to necrosis of the membranous labyrinth and an irreversible loss of vestibular and auditory function.[5]

Intracranial Complications of Otitic Infections

Chronic infection involving the perilabyrinthine bone may extend into the apical regions of the petrous bone, producing *petrositis.* Petrositis often presents as Gradenigo's syndrome, consisting of (1) otitis media, (2) paralysis of the ipsilateral lateral rectus muscle from involvement of the abducens nerve as it crosses the petrous bone, and (3) pain behind the ipsilateral eye from involvement of the trigeminal ganglion in the semilunar fossa. The syndrome may be associated with vertigo and hearing loss from either concomitant erosion of the bony labyrinth or involvement of the VIII nerve in its bony canal.

The most common intracranial complication of otitic infections is *extradural abscess,* a collection of pus between the dura mater and bone of the middle or posterior fossa.[5] The dura mater is usually an effective barrier, and the infection remains localized outside the nervous system. Rarely, spread of the infection across the dura results in *thrombophlebitis of the lateral venous sinus, subdural abscess, meningitis,* or *brain abscess,* or both.

Otitis externa may become a debilitating disease in elderly diabetic patients, producing so-called *malignant external otitis.*[6] Infection with Pseudomonas aeruginosa invades the junction of the cartilaginous and osseous portions of the external auditory canal and spreads to the temporo-occipital bones. The most common neurologic sequella is involvement of the facial nerve in the facial canal or at the stylomastoid foramen.[7] Hearing loss and vertigo from involvement of the VIII nerve are also common symptoms. Occasionally, multiple cranial nerves are compressed extradurally, and in rare cases the infection spreads across the dura to produce purulent meningitis.

Viral Labyrinthitis

Viral labyrinthitis may be part of a systemic viral illness, such as an upper respiratory tract infection, measles, mumps, and infectious mononucleosis, or it may be an isolated infection of the labyrinth without systemic involvement. Viruses probably reach the labyrinth via the systemic circulation. Although the infecting agent is rarely identified, substantial pathologic evidence exists that the sudden onset of hearing loss and vertigo can be caused by an acute isolated viral infection of the labyrinth.[5,8] The pathologic findings of atrophy of the organ of Corti

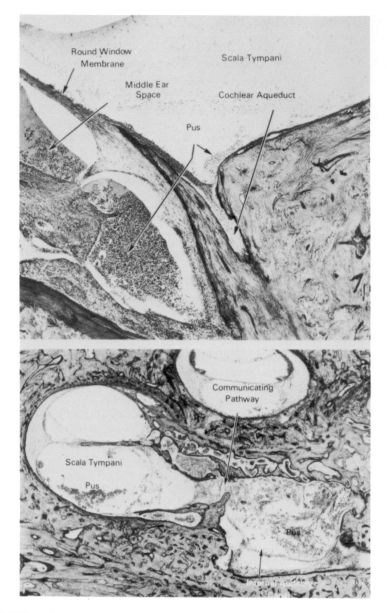

FIGURE 49. Histopathologic sections of the temporal bone from a patient with pneumococcal otitis media, labyrinthitis, and meningitis. Polymorphonuclear leukocytes fill the cochlear aqueduct (A) and the internal auditory canal (B), the two potential communicating pathways between the inner ear and the cerebrospinal fluid. Death occurred 3 days after the onset of meningeal symptoms and signs. (From Schucknecht, HF: *Pathology of the Ear.* Harvard University Press, Cambridge, MA, 1974, with permission.)

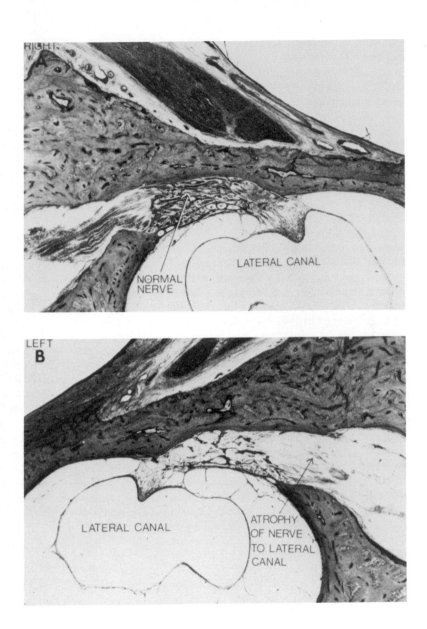

FIGURE 50. Histopathologic sections of the temporal bones from a patient with a left viral vestibular neuritis. (A) Normal nerve to the right horizontal semicircular canal; (B) atrophic nerve to the same canal on the left. Patient had three recurrent episodes of severe vertigo, nausea, and vomiting at age 55 and died of a myocardial infarction at age 71. (From Schuknecht, HF and Kitamuha, K: *Vestibular neuritis.* Ann Otol Rhinol Laryngol 90 (Suppl)78:1, 1981, with permission).

and atrophy of the vestibular end organs are similar to those seen with labyrinthitis associated with well-documented viral illnesses (such as mumps or measles). In such cases the vasculature remains intact and the cochlear and vestibular neuronal population is unaffected. As a general rule, a sudden onset of hearing loss and vertigo in an otherwise healthy patient is likely due to a viral labyrinthitis.

Viral Neuritis

One of the most common clinical neurotologic syndromes at any age is the acute onset of prolonged vertigo, nausea, and vomiting (lasting days) unassociated with auditory or neurologic symptoms. Most of these patients gradually improve over one to two weeks, but some develop recurrent episodes. A large percentage of such patients report an upper respiratory tract illness within one to two weeks prior to the onset of vertigo. This syndrome frequently occurs in epidemics (epidemic vertigo), may affect several members of the same family, and erupts more commonly in the spring and early summer.[9] All of these factors suggest a viral origin, but attempts to isolate an agent have been unsuccessful, except for occasional findings of a herpes zoster infection.[10,11] Pathologic studies showing atrophy of one or more vestibular nerve trunks, with or without atrophy of their associated sense organs, support a vestibular nerve site and probably viral etiology for this syndrome (i.e., *vestibular neuritis*) (Fig. 50).[12] Sudden unilateral hearing loss is another common clinical syndrome that is probably due to viral involvement of the auditory nerve *(acoustic neuritis)* in most cases.[13]

An example of a well-defined viral neuritis of the VII and VIII cranial nerves is *herpes zoster oticus.* With this condition the patient initially develops a deep, burning pain in the ear, followed a few days later by a vesicular eruption in the external auditory canal and concha (Fig. 51).[14] At some time after the onset of pain, either before or after the vesicular eruption, the patient may develop hearing loss, vertigo, and facial weakness. These symptoms may occur singly or collectively. The pathologic findings in patients with herpes zoster oticus consist of perivascular, perineural, and intraneural round cell infiltration in the VII, and in both divisions of the VIII nerve.[15]

Syphilitic Infections

Both congenital and acquired syphilitic infections produce labyrinthitis as a latent manifestation.[16] The congenital variety is approximately three times as common as the acquired variety. The time of onset of congenital syphilitic labyrinthitis can be anywhere from the first to seventh decades, with the peak incidence occurring in the fourth and fifth decades; acquired syphilitic labyrinthitis rarely occurs before the fourth decade and has a peak incidence in the fifth and sixth decades. The congenital variety is often associated with other stigmata of congenital syphilis, such as interstitial keratitis (Fig. 52), Hutchinson's teeth, saddle nose, frontal bossing, and rhagades. The natural history of syphilitic

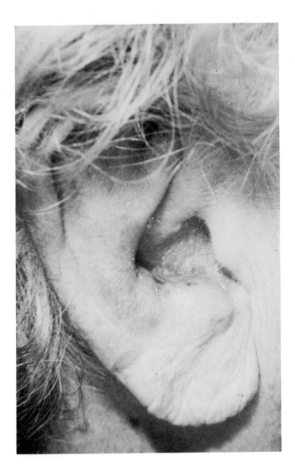

FIGURE 51. Vesicles in the external auditory canal in a patient with herpes zoster oticus. (Courtesy Rinaldo Canalis, M.D., Head and Neck Surgery, UCLA).

labyrinthitis is a slow relentless progression to profound or total bilateral loss of vestibular and auditory function. This progression is marked by episodes of sudden deafness and vertigo, and fluctuation in the magnitude of hearing loss and tinnitus. The pathologic changes in the labyrinth are similar in the congenital and acquired variety, consisting of inflammatory infiltration of the membranous labyrinth and osteitis of all three layers of the otic capsule.[5] A combination of hydrops of the membranous labyrinth and atrophy of cochlear and vestibular end organs resembles the pathologic findings in idiopathic Meniere's syndrome (see Fig. 59).

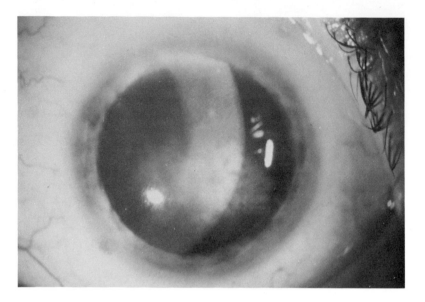

FIGURE 52. Interstitial keratitis. Dense white opacities in the stroma of the cornea stand out against the dark background of the dilated pupil. Wide beam of the slit-lamp illuminates opacities in the central area of the cornea. Milder cases can be identified only with the slit lamp. (Courtesy Robert Yee, M.D., Ophthalmology, UCLA).

VASCULAR DISORDERS

Vertebrobasilar Insufficiency

Vertebrobasilar insufficiency (VBI) is a common cause of vertigo in the elderly. Whether the vertigo originates from ischemia of the labyrinth, brainstem, or both structures is not always clear, since the blood supply to the labyrinth, VIII nerve, and vestibular nuclei originates from the same source, the vertebrobasilar circulation[17] (Fig. 53). As indicated in Chapter 2, the internal auditory artery, usually a branch of the anterior inferior cerebellar artery, supplies the VIII nerve and labyrinth. The anterior inferior cerebellar artery also supplies the rostral part of the vestibular nuclei, while the posterior inferior cerebellar artery supplies the caudal part of the vestibular nuclei.

Vertigo with VBI is abrupt in onset, usually lasting several minutes, and is frequently associated with nausea and vomiting. Associated symptoms resulting from ischemia in the remaining territory supplied by the posterior circulation include visual illusions and hallucinations, drop attacks and weakness, visceral sensations, visual field defects, diplopia, and headaches. These symptoms occur in episodes either in combination with the vertigo or in isolation. Vertigo may

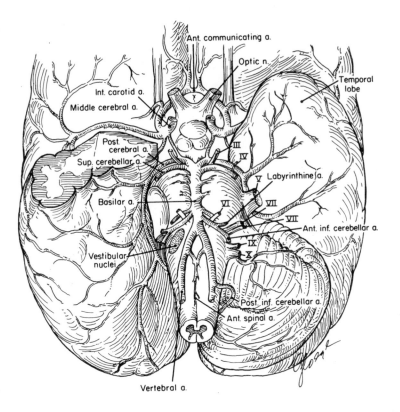

FIGURE 53. Vertebrobasilar circulation. Stippled area denotes location of the vestibular nuclei. In addition to the brainstem, labyrinths, and cerebellum, the vertebrobasilar circulation supplies the inferomedial part of the temporal lobes (including the hypocampus) and the occipital lobes via the posterior cerebral arteries. The latter accounts for the frequent occurrence of visual symptoms with vertebrobasilar insufficiency.

be an isolated initial symptom of VBI, but repeated episodes of vertigo without other symptoms should suggest another diagnosis.[18]

VBI is usually caused by atherosclerosis of the subclavian, vertebral, and basilar arteries.[19] Areas with a predilection for atherosclerotic plaques are shown in Figure 54. Occasionally, episodes of VBI are precipitated by postural hypotension, Stokes-Adams attacks, or mechanical compression from cervical spondylosis.[20] The patient whose angiogram is shown in Figure 55 had a complete blockage of the right vertebral artery near its origin, and compression of the left vertebral artery by osteoarthritic spurs. He developed episodic vertigo, diplopia, and generalized weakness when he turned his head to the right (resulting in complete blockage of the left vertebral artery). Rarely, occlusion or stenosis of the subclavian or innominate arteries just proximal to the origin of the vertebral artery results in the so-called *subclavian steal syndrome*. In this syn-

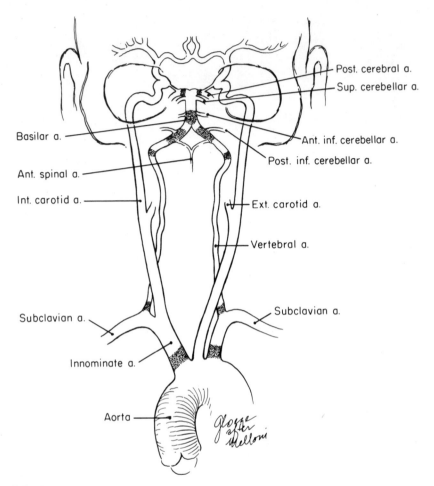

Post. cerebral a.
Sup. cerebellar a.
Basilar a.
Ant. inf. cerebellar a.
Post. inf. cerebellar a.
Ant. spinal a.
Int. carotid a.
Ext. carotid a.
Vertebral a.
Subclavian a.
Subclavian a.
Innominate a.
Aorta

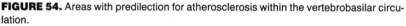

FIGURE 54. Areas with predilection for atherosclerosis within the vertebrobasilar circulation.

drome, VBI results from a siphoning of blood down the vertebral artery from the basilar system to supply the upper extremities. Vertigo and other symptoms of VBI are precipitated by exercise of the upper extremities.

Migraine

Vertigo can precede or accompany the headache of both classic and common migraine. Bickerstaff reported an unusual variety of migraine in which the aura consisted entirely of posterior fossa symptoms such as vertigo, ataxia, dysarthria, and tinnitus, along with positive visual phenomena in both visual fields.[21]

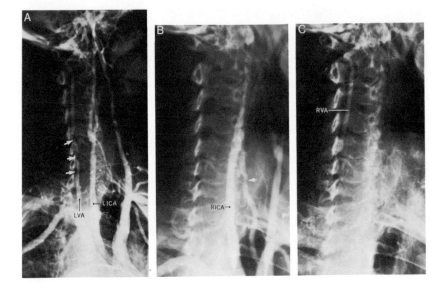

FIGURE 55. Angiogram from a patient with vertebrobasilar insufficiency. In the left lateral projection (A), the left vertebral artery (LVA) is indented with osteoarthritic spurs (arrows). In the right lateral projection (B and C), the right vertebral artery (RVA) initially does not fill (B), but then fills via retrograde flow (C). LICA—left internal carotid artery, RICA—right internal carotid artery.

These aura symptoms lasted from 2 to 45 minutes and were followed by a throbbing unilateral occipital headache. Between attacks many of the patients experienced classical migraine episodes, and over the years the atypical episodes were replaced with more typical ones. Twenty-six of the 34 cases reported were of adolescent girls, and the attacks were strikingly related to their menstrual periods. Bickerstaff postulated that the aura phenomena were secondary to vasoconstriction in the vertebrobasilar system, and called the syndrome *basilar artery migraine.* He further postulated that patients with vertigo as part of a more usual migraine aura (e.g., visual scotoma) develop ischemia simultaneously in the distribution of several vessels, including the basilar artery. A more recent report documented the frequent occurrence of both vestibular paresis and directional preponderance to caloric stimulation in patients with basilar artery migraine.[22]

Benign Paroxysmal Vertigo of Childhood

In young children the manifestations of migraine are more protean and headache is not always prominent. So-called *migraine equivalents* may present as cyclical vomiting, attacks of abdominal pain, and episodes of vertigo or dysequilibrium. As the child matures these nonspecific and often puzzling symptoms cease, and are supplanted by more typical paroxysmal head pain. Basser reported a common clinical disorder in children under the age of 4, which he called benign paroxysmal vertigo.[23] This syndrome was characterized by brief episodes of vertigo (usually lasting seconds, rarely more than a few minutes), often accompanied by pallor, sweating, and vomiting that recurred several times a week to once a year, and then ceased spontaneously. The etiology of benign paroxysmal vertigo is unknown, although most authors suspect a vascular disturbance affecting the posterior cerebral circulation.[24] Follow-up studies of patients with typical benign paroxysmal vertigo of childhood indicate that 50 percent subsequently develop classical migraine.[25]

Labyrinthine Infarction

Since the labyrinthine artery divides into a cochlear and vestibular branch, there is an anatomic substrate for isolated infarction of either the auditory or vestibular labyrinth (see Fig. 7). The former would result in sudden unilateral deafness, while the latter would produce an acute vestibular syndrome. How often such vascular events occur is disputed, owing primarily to lack of pathologic confirmation.[26] This diagnosis must be kept in mind, however, in elderly subjects with known atherosclerotic vascular disease, particularly if they have a prior history of occlusive disease in other cerebral arteries. More commonly, labyrinthine infarction is associated with brain stem and cerebellar infarction as part of the anterior inferior cerebellar artery syndrome (see below).

Cogan's Syndrome

Patients with Cogan's syndrome present with interstitial keratitis, episodic vertigo, tinnitus, and deafness.[27] These patients have no clinical or laboratory evidence of syphilis or any other specific disease. The onset of symptoms is abrupt, with severe vertigo, nausea, vomiting, and hearing loss. The hearing loss may initially be unilateral, but within a few weeks to months both sides are involved. The eye and ear manifestations may occur simultaneously, or the onset of one may be delayed for several months. Cogan's syndrome may also be part of a general systemic illness.[28] Five reported cases occurred in patients with well-documented polyarteritis nodosa; one patient had proven sarcoidosis. In many other cases described in the literature clinical manifestations suggested collagen vascular disease. Pathologic studies of the temporal bone are sparse and have not shown localized vasculitis, even in patients with prominent vasculitis in other organs.[29,30] The most consistent finding has been diffuse degeneration of all neural elements in the inner ear.

Brainstem Infarction

Neurotologic symptoms are common with infarction of the lateral brainstem or cerebellum, or both. The zone of infarction producing *Wallenberg's syndrome*

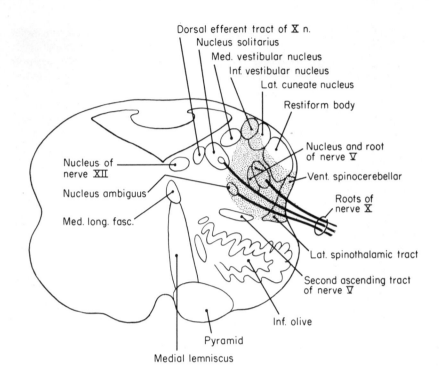

Dorsal efferent tract of X n.
Nucleus solitarius
Med. vestibular nucleus
Inf. vestibular nucleus
Lat. cuneate nucleus
Restiform body
Nucleus and root of nerve V
Vent. spinocerebellar
Roots of nerve X
Nucleus of nerve XII
Nucleus ambiguus
Med. long. fasc.
Lat. spinothalamic tract
Second ascending tract of nerve V
Inf. olive
Pyramid
Medial lemniscus

FIGURE 56. Cross-section of the medulla illustrating the zone of infarction with Wallenberg's syndrome (stippled area).

consists of a wedge of the dorsolateral medulla just posterior to the inferior olive supplied by the posteroinferior cerebellar artery (Fig. 56). It usually occurs from occlusion of the ipsilateral vertebral artery, and infrequently from occlusion of the posteroinferior cerebellar artery.[31] Characteristic symptoms include vertigo, ipsilateral facial pain, diplopia, dysphagia, and dysphonia. Some patients develop a prominent motor disturbance that causes their bodies and extremities to deviate toward the lesion side, as if being pulled by a strong external force.[32] This so-called lateropulsion also affects the oculomotor system, producing excessively large saccades directed toward the side of the lesion, while saccades away from the side of the lesion are abnormally small.[33] Ischemia in the distribution of the anteroinferior cerebellar artery usually results in infarction of the dorsolateral pontomedullary region and the inferolateral cerebellum *(lateral pontomedullary syndrome)*.[34] Since the labyrinthine artery arises from the anteroinferior cerebellar artery, approximately 80 percent of the time infarction of the membranous labyrinth is a common accompaniment. Severe vertigo, nausea, and vomiting are the initial and most prominent symptoms. Other associated symptoms include unilateral hearing loss, tinnitus, facial paralysis, and cerebellar asynergy.

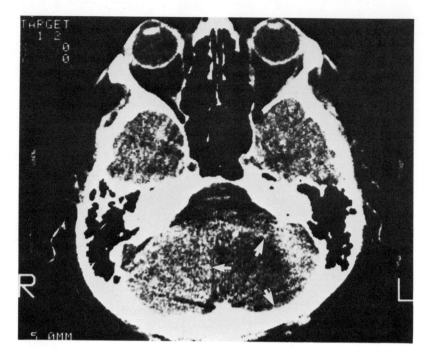

FIGURE 57. C-T scan of the posterior fossa illustrating a cerebellar infarction (demarcated by arrows).

Cerebellar Infarction

In some instances occlusion of the vertebral artery, the posteroinferior cerebellar artery, or the anteroinferior cerebellar artery results in infarction confined to the posteroinferior cerebellar hemisphere without accompanying brainstem involvement (Fig. 57).[35,36] The initial symptoms are severe vertigo, vomiting, and ataxia, and since typical brainstem signs do not occur, the mistaken diagnosis of an acute peripheral labyrinthine disorder might be made. The key differential point is the finding on examination of prominent ipsilateral cerebellar signs, particularly ipsilateral extremity and gait ataxia and gaze-evoked nystagmus. After a latent interval of 24 to 96 hours, some patients develop progressive brainstem dysfunction owing to compression by a swollen cerebellum.[36]

Intralabyrinthine Hemorrhage

Intralabyrinthine hemorrhage occurs mainly in patients with an underlying bleeding diathesis. Leukemia is the most common disorder associated with labyrinthine hemorrhage.[37] Such patients experience sudden onset of unilateral deafness and severe vertigo. Pathologic examination of the inner ear reveals hemorrhage into the perilymphatic space, with smaller focal hemorrhages in the endolymphatic space. The vestibular and cochlear end organs, although morphologically intact, are rendered nonfunctional, apparently from altered fluid chemistry. A similar intralabyrinthine hemorrhage may follow a blow to the head without the occurrence of bony fracture.[5]

Cerebellar Hemorrhage

Spontaneous intraparenchymal hemorrhage into the brainstem and cerebellum causes multiple neurologic symptoms and signs that often progress to coma and death (Fig. 58). In the vast majority of patients the cause of the hemorrhage is hypertensive vascular disease.[38] The initial symptoms of cerebellar hemorrhage are often vertigo, nausea, vomiting, headache, and inability to stand or walk.[39,40] This early syndrome is distinguished from more benign labyrinthine disorders by the finding on neurologic examination of nuchal rigidity and prominent cerebellar signs. Obstructive hydrocephalus and brainstem compression typically follow within hours to days of the acute hemorrhage. Approximately 50 percent of patients lose consciousness within 24 hours of the initial symptoms, and 75 percent become comatose within one week of onset. The condition is often fatal unless surgical decompression is performed. The earlier the syndrome is recognized, the more likely that surgery will be successful. Once patients become comatose, almost none survive.[41] Midline cerebellar hemorrhage is particularly difficult to diagnose because it produces bilateral signs and generally runs a more fulminant course than lateralized hemorrhage.

Brainstem Hemorrhage

In contrast to cerebellar hemorrhage, spontaneous hemorrhage into the brainstem is associated with rapid loss of consciousness, usually without prodromal symptoms. Intrapontine hemorrhage results in rapid onset of coma, flaccid quadriplegia, loss of horizontal eye movements, and pinpoint reactive pupils. Hemorrhage into the medulla is associated with rapid cardiorespiratory failure and death.

MENIERE'S SYNDROME (ENDOLYMPHATIC HYDROPS)

Meniere's syndrome is characterized by fluctuating hearing loss and tinnitus, episodic vertigo, and a sensation of fullness or pressure in the ear. Typically the patient develops a sensation of fullness and pressure, along with decreased hearing and tinnitus in one ear. Vertigo rapidly follows, reaching a maximum intensity within minutes, and then slowly subsiding over the next several hours. The patient is usually left with a sense of unsteadiness and dizziness for days after the acute vertiginous episode. In the early stages the hearing loss is com-

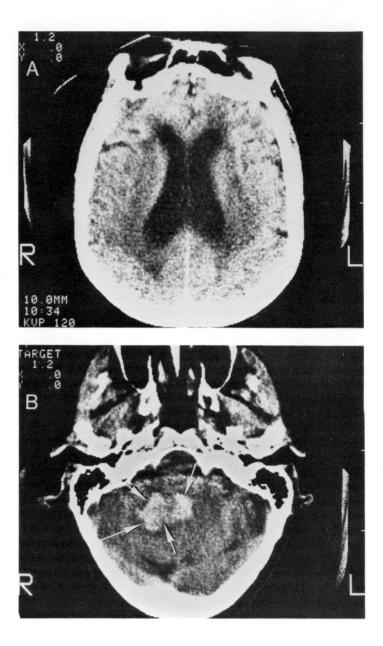

FIGURE 58. C-T scans showing hydrocephalus (A) caused by a cerebellar hemorrhage; (B) arrows outline hemorrhage.

pletely reversible, but in later stages a residual hearing loss remains (see Fig. 41).

Variations from this characteristic profile occur, particularly in the early stages of the disease process, but the diagnosis remains uncertain unless the combination of fluctuating hearing loss and vertigo occurs. Although so-called vestibular Meniere's and cochlear Meniere's have been proposed as variations of the classic syndrome, clinicopathologic correlation of isolated vestibular and auditory disorders with selective endolymphatic hydrops of the vestibular and auditory labyrinth is lacking. Some patients with well-documented Meniere's syndrome experience abrupt episodes of falling to the ground without loss of consciousness or associated neurologic symptoms. They may initially feel that some external force pushed them over. These episodes have been called otolithic catastrophes, since they are thought to be due to sudden stimulation of the otoliths.[42]

The main pathologic finding in patients with Meniere's syndrome is distention of the entire endolymphatic system (Fig. 59).[5,43] The membranous labyrinth progressively dilates until the saccular wall makes contact with the stapes footplate and the cochlear duct occupies the entire vestibular scala. The cochlear and vestibular end organs and nerves show minimal pathologic changes. Membranous labyrinth herniations and ruptures are common, the latter frequently involving Reissner's membrane and the walls of the saccule, utricle, and ampullae.[44] Occasionally, a rupture is followed by complete collapse of the membranous labyrinth.

Several diseases are known to produce Meniere's syndrome, but in the majority of cases the cause is unknown. Bacterial, viral, and syphilitic labyrinthitis (see Infection) can all lead to endolymphatic hydrops and typical symptoms and signs of Meniere's syndrome. In this case hydrops results from damage to fluid resorptive mechanisms owing to inflammation and scarring.

Patients with idiopathic Meniere's syndrome frequently have a positive family history (in some reports as high as 50 percent), suggesting genetic predisposing factors.[45] Several investigators have produced endolymphatic hydrops in animals by either blocking the endolymphatic duct, or destroying the endolymphatic sac.[5] This led to a series of surgical procedures designed to open the endolymphatic duct in patients with idiopathic Meniere's syndrome. Widely disparate results for these surgical procedures appear in the literature.[1,46]

Although the pathologic changes have been well described, the mechanism for the fluctuating symptoms and signs of Meniere's syndrome are not well understood. A leading theory is that the episodes of hearing loss and vertigo are caused by ruptures in the membranes separating endolymph from perilymph, producing a sudden increase in potassium concentration in the latter.[47] As the potassium is slowly cleared over several hours, the symptoms and signs subside. Another possible explanation is mechanical deformation of the end organ that is reversible as the endolymphatic pressure decreases.[48] The sudden falling attacks seen in patients with Meniere's syndrome are most likely due to

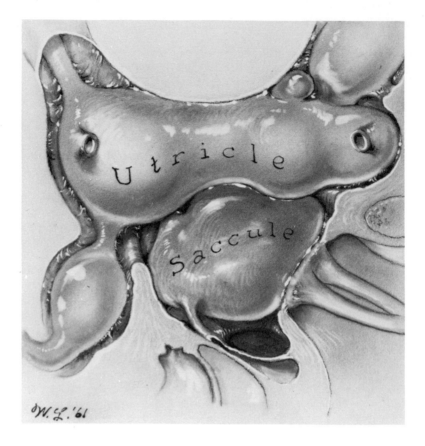

FIGURE 59. Dilated membranous labyrinth in Meniere's syndrome. The drawing was made from a three-dimensional model developed from serial sections of the ear of a patient with Meniere's syndrome. (From Schuknecht, HF: *Pathology of the Ear.* Harvard University Press, Cambridge, MA, 1974, with permission).

deformation or displacement of one of the otolith organs by a rapid change in inner ear pressure.

DEGENERATIVE DISORDERS OF THE LABYRINTH

Benign Paroxysmal Positional Vertigo

Patients with benign paroxysmal positional vertigo develop brief episodes of vertigo (30 seconds) with position change, typically when turning over in bed, bending over and straightening up, or extending the neck to look up. Benign paroxysmal positional vertigo can result from head injury, viral labyrinthitis, and vascular occlusion, or it may occur as an isolated symptom of unknown cause.[49,50,51] The latter is particularly common in the elderly. This syndrome is important to recognize, since in the vast majority of patients the symptoms spontaneously remit within six months of onset. The diagnosis rests on finding characteristic paroxysmal positional nystagmus after a rapid change from the sitting to head-hanging position (see Positional Nystagmus, Chapter 7).

Studies of the temporal bones of a few patients with typical benign paroxysmal positional nystagmus have revealed basophilic deposits on the cupulae of the posterior canals (Fig. 60).[52] These deposits were present only on one side, the side that was undermost when paroxysmal positional nystagmus and vertigo were induced. These cupular basophilic deposits are apparently otoconia released from a degenerating utricular macule. The otoconia settle on the cupula of the posterior canal (situated directly under the utricular macule), causing it to become heavier than the surrounding endolymph. When the patient moves from the sitting to head-hanging position (provocative test for paroxysmal positional nystagmus), the posterior canal moves from an inferior to superior position, a utriculofugal displacement of the cupula occurs, and a burst of nystagmus is produced. The latency before nystagmus onset could be due to the period of time required for the otoconial mass to be displaced and fatigability may be caused by the dispersing of particles in the endolymph. Consistent with this theory, the burst of rotatory paroxysmal positional nystagmus is in the plane of the posterior canal of the "down" ear, with the fast component directed upward (toward the forehead) as would be predicted from ampullofugal stimulation of the posterior canal.[51] Additional support for this concept has come from reports showing disappearance of fatigable paroxysmal positonal nystagmus after the ampullary nerve has been sectioned from the posterior canal on the diseased side.[53]

Effects of Aging on the Auditory and Vestibular Systems

As with all other sensory systems, the auditory and vestibular systems undergo numerous changes with aging.[54,55] There is a gradual loss of sensory cells and primary afferent neurons, accompanied by loss of otoconia from the macules (particularly in the saccule) and accumulation of lipofucsin granules in the remaining sensory, ganglion, and supporting cells. Because the functional role of the vestibular system overlaps that of the proprioceptive and visual systems, a gradual loss of vestibular function with aging could easily be masked. By contrast, degenerative changes with aging in the nearby auditory system have clear clinical effects.

The bilateral hearing loss commonly associated with advancing age is called *presbycusis.* Presbycusis is not a distinct disease entity, but rather represents multiple effects of aging on the auditory system.[5] Presbycusis may include conductive and central dysfunction, although the most consistent effect of aging is on the sensory cells and neurons of the cochlea. The typical audiogram

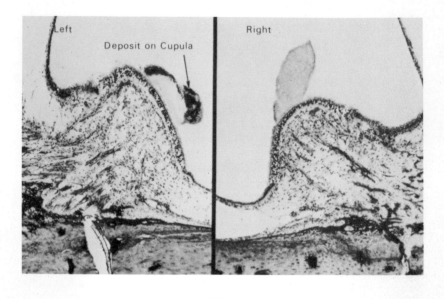

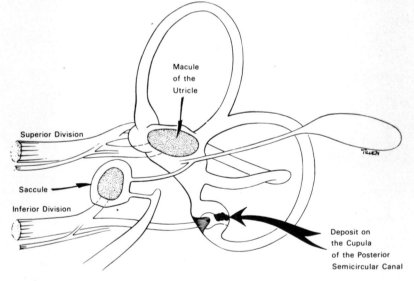

FIGURE 60. *(Top)* Histopathologic section through the cristae of the posterior semicircular canals of a patient who exhibited typical benign paroxysmal positional vertigo and nystagmus in the head-hanging left position prior to death from unrelated causes. Attached to the cupula of the left posterior canal is a granular, basophilic staining deposit. *(Bottom)* This drawing illustrates that when the head is erect, the ampulla of the posterior semicircular canal is directly below the macule of the utricle. (From Schuknecht, HF: *Pathology of the Ear.* Harvard University Press, Cambridge, MA, 1974, with permission).

of presbycusis is a symmetrical hearing loss gradually sloping downward with increasing frequency (see Fig. 41). The most consistent pathology associated with presbycusis is a degeneration of sensory cells and nerve fibers at the base of the cochlea.[5]

Surprisingly, function studies of the vestibulo-ocular reflex (both caloric and rotatory tests) do not consistently show a gradual decline in response with aging.[56,57] Occasional elderly normal subjects have hyperresponsiveness. Apparently two separate phenomena are occurring with aging—loss of central inhibitory control and loss of end organ function. The balance between these two changes determines the response of the vestibulo-ocular reflex. Based on the discussion of the pathophysiology of vestibular symptoms in Chapter 5, a gradual symmetrical loss of vestibular end organ function would not be expected to produce vertigo, but it would produce visual distortion and gait imbalance owing to loss of vestibulo-ocular and vestibulospinal reflex function.

Clinical experience has shown that *dysequilibrium* is a common symptom in elderly patients. Such patients usually complain of severe unsteadiness when walking, but minimal or no dysequilibrium when sitting or standing. Their gait is characterized by hesitancy, with frequent side steps and a fixed head position to gain optimum advantage of visual points of reference. Typically, ambulation is most difficult in a darkened room. All of these features suggest that loss of vestibular function is an important component of their disequilibrium. Furthermore, since parallel degenerative changes occur with aging in other sensory systems and within the central nervous system itself, degenerative changes in the vestibular end organs are even more important (i.e., the concept of *multisensory dizziness*).

TUMORS

Primary Carcinoma

Epidermoid carcinomas arise from epidermal cells of the auricle, external auditory canal, or the middle ear and mastoid. The prognosis is good for tumors confined to the auricle and external canal, but not for those invading the middle ear and mastoid. The latter are frequently associated with prominent neurotologic symptoms that typically include vertigo, hearing loss, pain, otorrhea, mastoid swelling, and facial paralysis.[5,58] The tumor is frequently visible in the external canal, and erosion of the temporal bone is apparent on x-ray examination.

Metastatic Carcinoma

Metastatic involvement of the temporal bone occurs with several different tumor types, but apparently because of the enchondral layer's resistance, neoplasms rarely invade the bony labyrinth. The most common site of origin for metastatic tumors in order of frequency is: breast, kidney, lung, stomach, larynx, prostate, and thyroid gland.[59] The internal auditory canal is a frequent site of metastatic tumor growth within the temporal bone. From this site tumor cells destroy the VII and VIII nerves and extend into the inner ear or into the cerebellopontine angle. Irregular destruction of bone by the rapidly growing tumor is usually apparent on x-ray examination. Metastatic tumors from the breast and prostate commonly incite new bone formation.

Glomus Body Tumors

Glomus body tumors are the most common tumor of the middle ear, and next to acoustic neuromas are the most common tumor of the temporal bone. Glomus tumors arise in the glomera of the chemoreceptor system, which may be found along the vagus nerve, glossopharyngeal nerve, Jacobson's nerve (tympanic branch of IX), and the nerve of Arnold (postauricular branch of X). The most common tumor sites are the glomus jugulare (jugular bulb), glomus tympanicum (middle ear), and the glomus vagale (along the course of the vagus nerve). Glomus vagale and jugulare tumors often involve the labyrinth and cranial nerves, while glomus tympanicum tumors usually produce only local symptoms because of the tumor bulk in the middle ear, that is, conductive hearing loss and pulsatile tinnitus (see Fig. 3C).[60] Invasion of the labyrinth is an uncommon but serious prognostic sign and is often associated with extension to the petrous apex and into the middle and posterior fossa.

Acoustic Neuroma

Acoustic neuromas (vestibular schwannomas) usually begin on the vestibular nerve in the internal auditory canal, producing symptoms by compressing the nerves in the narrow confines of the canal (Fig. 61). As the tumor enlarges it protrudes through the internal auditory canal producing a funnel-shaped erosion of the bone surrounding the canal, stretching adjacent nerve roots over the surface of the mass, and deforming the brainstem and cerebellum. Acoustic neuromas account for approximately 10 percent of intracranial tumors and over 75 percent of cerebellopontine angle tumors.[61,62] By far the most common symptoms associated with acoustic neuromas are slowly progressive hearing loss and tinnitus from compression of the cochlear nerve. Occasionally, an acute hearing loss occurs apparently from compression of the labyrinthine vasculature. Vertigo occurs in less than 20 percent of patients, but approximately 50 percent complain of imbalance or dysequilibrium. Large tumors may compress the VII and V cranial nerves, producing facial weakness and numbness respectively. Involvement of the VI, IX, X, XI, and XII nerves occurs only in the late stages of disease with massive tumors. Large acoustic neuromas may also produce increased intracranial pressure from obstruction of cerebrospinal fluid outflow.

Bilateral acoustic neuromas occur in approximately 5 percent of patients with neurofibromatosis, and occasionally are the only manifestation of the disease.[63] A young patient with a unilateral acoustic neuroma and a family history of neurofibromatosis has a high probability of developing a second acoustic neuroma on the opposite side. *Facial nerve schwannomas* often begin in the

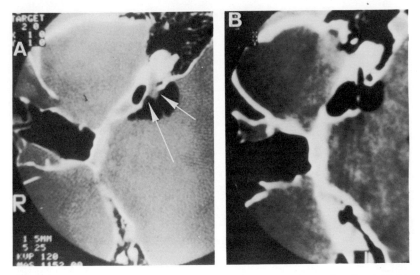

FIGURE 61. Air C-T scan showing a small acoustic neuroma (arrows) on the right side (A), and normal internal auditory canal on the left side (B).

internal auditory canal, producing slowly progressive hearing loss similar to an acoustic neuroma. Early involvement of the facial nerve (i.e., facial weakness) is a useful distinguishing feature.

Other Cerebellopontine Angle Tumors

Next to acoustic neuromas the most common primary tumors of the cerebellopontine angle are meningiomas and epidermoid cysts.[61] *Meningiomas* arise from arachnoid fibroblasts, usually near the sigmoid and petrosal sinuses on the petrous pyramid.[64] The lobulated variety is more common than the flat (en plaque) type. Meningiomas are frequently calcified, and induce osteoblastic reaction in adjacent bone. Both of these features are visible on routine x-rays. *Epidermoid cysts* arise from congenital inclusion rests in the area of the petrous apex.[65] They slowly enlarge to fill the cerebellopontine angle, stretching nearby cranial nerves and compressing the brainstem (Fig. 62). In addition to the usual symptoms and signs of tumors in this region, hemifacial spasm is a frequent early symptom.

DEVELOPMENTAL DISORDERS

Congenital Malformations of the Inner Ear

Congenital malformations of the inner ear can result from abnormal genetic or intrauterine factors. Genetically determined deafness may be present at birth,

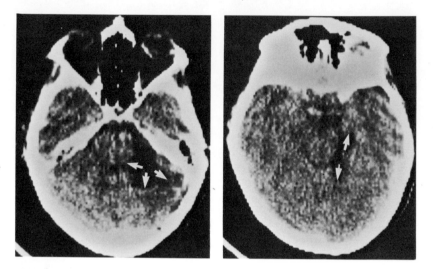

FIGURE 62. C-T scans of the posterior fossa showing an epidermoid cyst in the right cerebellar pontine angle (arrows).

or it may become manifest years after birth as the normally developed inner ear structures deteriorate.[66,67] In approximately one-third of cases there is a clearly defined syndrome, but in the majority of cases the diagnosis of *hereditary deafness* rests on the finding of a positive family history. *Alport's syndrome* is a sex-linked inherited sensorineural deafness associated with interstitial nephritis. *Waardenburg's syndrome* is a dominantly inherited sensorineural deafness associated with lateral displacement of the medial canthae, hyperplastic high nasal root, hyperplasia of the medial portions of the eyebrows, partial or total heterochromia irides, and circumscribed albinism of the frontal head hair (white forelock). A combination of recessively inherited retinitis pigmentosa and sensorineural deafness is known as *Usher's syndrome.* All of these disorders may have associated bilateral loss of vestibular function. Although congenital deafness is usually recognized during infancy, congenital vestibular impairment is not, because the manifestations are more subtle. Children learn to use other sensory information to compensate for vestibular loss, and usually appear normal on standard developmental tests.

Intrauterine factors resulting in maldevelopment of the inner ear include infection, toxic, metabolic, and endocrine disorders, and anoxia associated with Rh incompatibility and difficult deliveries.[5] As many as 70 percent of mothers who acquire *rubella* during the first trimester of pregnancy will produce a child with some degree of hearing loss.[68,69] Impaired hearing is more common than impaired vestibular function, apparently because of the longer critical developmental period of the cochlea (see Development of the Labyrinth, Chapter 2).

After conclusion of the first trimester the risk is significantly less, but the infant's formed inner ear can still become infected from a maternal rubella infection. If the maternal infection occurs in the first six weeks of gestation, malformations of the eyes, cardiovascular system, and brain are also common.

The first pathologic study of an inner ear congenital malformation was reported by Mondini in 1791.[70,71] The *Mondini malformation* consists of subtotal development of the osseous and membranous labyrinth, with only the basal turn of the cochlea being completely formed. The endolymphatic duct system is dilated and the vestibular labyrinth is underdeveloped. This deformity occurs with many different syndromes, both hereditary and acquired, and is invariably associated with some (and often complete) loss of auditory and vestibular function. *Cochleosaccular dysgenesis,* initially described by Scheibe, consists of dysplasia of the cochlea and saccule, with a fully developed bony labyrinth and normal semicircular canals and utricle. The Scheibe deformity is frequently produced by congenital rubella, accounting for the relative sparing of vestibular function in many of these children. A rare deformity characterized by complete failure of development of the inner ear *(Michel deformity)* is associated with total loss of auditory and vestibular function. This deformity has been found in several patients with thalidomide anomalies of the ear.

Malformations of the Craniovertebral Junction

Bony malformations of the craniovertebral junction may be associated with the clinical complaints of vertigo, imbalance, and hearing loss. *Basilar impression* is a deformity of the base of the skull in which the bony rim of the foramen magnum is elevated into the cranial cavity. Cerebellar ataxia and damage to the lower cranial nerves result from cerebellar and brainstem compression. With the *Klippel-Feil syndrome,* the cervical vertebrae are fused into a single column of bone. A characteristic clinical triad includes short neck, low hairline, and limitation of neck movements. Many patients with this syndrome are deaf from birth. Pathologic examination of the temporal bone in one such patient reveals a vestigial inner ear having a rudimentary cystic cavity for a cochlea, and only one semicircular canal, incompletely formed.[72]

The *Arnold-Chiari malformation* is a developmental defect of the cervicomedullary junction not infrequently associated with vestibular symptoms. With this soft tissue malformation, the caudal brainstem and cerebellum are elongated and protrude downward into the cervical canal (Fig. 63). Most frequently the deformity manifests itself in the first few months of life, and is associated with hydrocephalus and other nervous system malformations. Less frequent, but more important to the neurotologist, are those cases in which the onset of symptoms and signs is delayed until adult life. These cases often present with subtle neurologic symptoms and signs, and are usually unassociated with other developmental defects. The most common neurologic symptom is slowly progressive unsteadiness of gait which the patient frequently describes as dizziness. Vertigo and hearing loss occur in less than 10 percent of patients.[73]

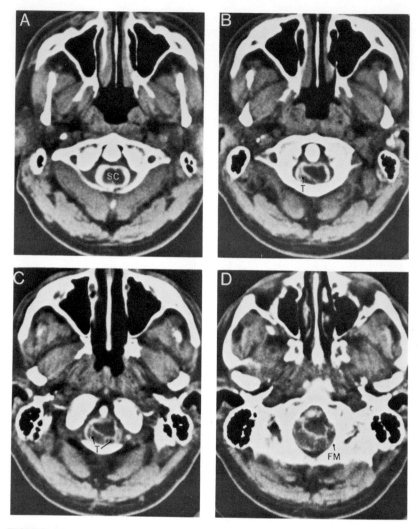

FIGURE 63. Metrizamine C-T scan sections ascending from C-2 (A) to the foramen magnum (D). Cerebellar tonsils surround and compress cervical-medullary junction. SC—spinal cord, T—tonsil, FM—foramen magnum.

TRAUMA

Temporal Bone Fracture

Longitudinal fractures of the temporal bone pass parallel to the anterior margin of the petrous pyramid, and usually extend from the region of the gasserian

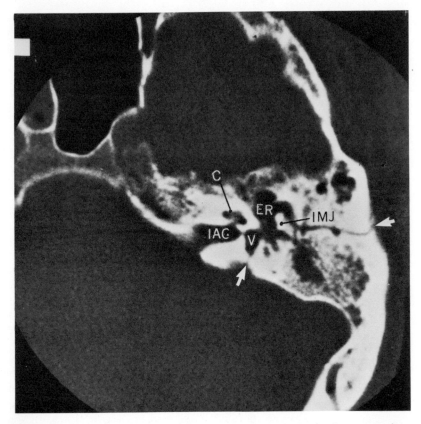

FIGURE 64. C-T scans of the temporal bone showing longitudinal and transverse fractures in the same patient (arrows). The longitudinal fracture crosses the middle ear, disrupting the ossicular chain, while the transverse fracture enters the vestibule, damaging the membranous labyrinth. C—cochlea, ER—epitympanic recess, IMJ—incudomalleal joint, V—vestibule, IAC—internal auditory canal. (Courtesy William Hanafee, M.D. and Sven Larson, M.D., Radiology, UCLA).

ganglion medially to the middle ear, and mastoid air cells laterally (Fig. 64).[5,74] Typically, the fracture line transverses the annulus tympanicus, lacerating the tympanic membrane, and producing a steplike deformity in the external auditory canal (see Fig. 3). Cerebrospinal and hemorrhagic otorrhea are common, and the combination of laceration of the tympanic membrane, ossicular damage, and hemotympanum produces a conductive hearing loss. Damage to the VII and VIII cranial nerves is infrequent.

By contrast, *transverse fractures* of the temporal bone run orthogonal to the long axis of the petrous pyramid, passing through the vestibule of the inner ear, tearing the membranous labyrinth and lacerating the vestibular and cochlear nerves (see Fig. 64). Complete loss of vestibular and cochlear function is the usual sequela, and the facial nerve is lacerated in approximately 50 percent of cases. Examination of the ear reveals hemotympanum, but bleeding from the ear occurs infrequently, since the tympanic membrane usually remains intact. CSF often fills the middle ear and drains through the eustachian tube into the nasopharynx. Meningitis is a late complication of both types of temporal bone fractures.

Labyrinthine Concussion

Vertigo, hearing loss, and tinnitus often follow a blow to the head that does not result in temporal bone fracture—so-called labyrinthine concussion.[75] Although protected by a bony capsule, the delicate labyrinthine membranes are susceptible to blunt trauma. Blows to the occipital or mastoid region are particularly likely to produce labyrinthine damage. Paradoxically, a blow that does not fracture the skull may produce more labyrinthine damage than one in which the forces are absorbed by an actual break in the bones. The most common vestibular symptom of head trauma is *positional vertigo.*[76] The patient develops sudden, brief attacks of vertigo and nystagmus, precipitated by changing head position typical of so-called benign paroxysmal positional vertigo. The trauma apparently dislodges otoconia from the utricular macule, which in turn settle on the cupula of the posterior semicircular canal (see Degenerative Disorders of the Labyrinth). The prognosis for patients with post-traumatic positional vertigo is good, with spontaneous remission occurring in most patients within six months, and almost always within two years of the head injury.[76,77]

Sudden deafness following a blow to the head, with or without associated vestibular symptoms, is often partially or completely reversible.[75] It is probably caused by intense acoustic stimulation from pressure waves created by the blow that are transmitted through the bone to the cochlea, just as pressure waves are transmitted from air through the conduction mechanism.[78] Supporting this suggestion, the pathologic changes in the cochlea produced by experimental head blows in animals are similar to those produced by intense airborne sound stimuli.[5]

Perilymph Fistula

Fistulae of the oval and round windows can result from impact noise, deep water diving, severe physical exertion, or blunt head injury without skull fracture.[5,79] The mechanism of the rupture is a sudden negative or positive pressure change in the middle ear, or a sudden increase in CSF pressure transmitted to the inner ear via the cochlear aqueduct and internal auditory canal (Fig. 65). Clinically, the rupture leads to the sudden onset of vertigo or hearing loss, or both. Surgical exploration of the middle ear is warranted when there is a clear-cut relationship between the onset of vertigo or hearing loss, or both, and either severe exertion, barometric change, head injury, or impact noise.

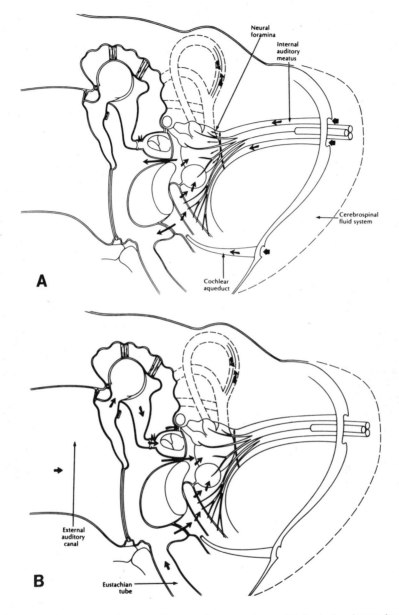

FIGURE 65. Causes of labyrinthine membrane ruptures. (A) Explosive forces from cerebrospinal fluid via the cochlear aqueduct or internal auditory canal; and (B) implosive forces from the middle ear, eustachian tube and external ear. (From Goodhill, V: *Ear Diseases, Deafness and Dizziness.* Harper and Row, Hagerstown, Md., 1979, with permission).

Otitic Barotrauma

So-called otitic barotrauma (aerotitis) is a traumatic inflammatory disorder of the middle ear caused by sudden severe negative pressure in the pneumatized spaces of the temporal bone.[5] The intense negative pressure results in medial displacement and stretching of the tympanic membrane, hyperemia, and edema, and ecchymosis of the mucous membranes of the middle ear, followed by transudation of fluid which may become sanguinous in severe cases. The main symptom is excruciating pain in the ear that gradually subsides over a period of hours. Occasionally, there is an associated conductive hearing loss owing to damage of the tympanic membrane and ossicular chain and, rarely, vertigo and sensorineural hearing loss, probably from rupture of the labyrinthine windows.[5,80] Otitic barotrauma typically occurs during descent from high altitudes, or during ascent from underwater diving. It is caused by failure of the eustachian tube to open sufficiently to permit the equalization of middle ear pressure.

Noise-Induced Hearing Loss

Noise-induced hearing loss is extremely common in our industrialized society. The loss almost always begins at 4000 Hz, and does not affect speech discrimination until late in the disease process.[81] With only a brief exposure to loud noise (hours to days), there may be only a temporary threshold shift, but with continued exposure permanent injury begins.[5,82] Damage to sensory cells is often confined to a small area at the base of the cochlea, centering around the area sensing 4000 Hz.

There are two main theories to explain the remarkable tendency for noise-induced injuries to involve this 8 to 10 millimeter region at the base of the cochlea.[5] The mechanical view holds that strong destructive forces develop owing to a "jet effect" at this particular region. The vascular theory maintains that this region is especially vulnerable to ischemia because it is at the juncture of the main cochlear artery and the cochlear ramus artery. Pathologic studies in patients with typical noise-induced hearing loss document a loss of hair cells between 5 to 10 millimeters from the base of the cochlea.[5] Electron microscopic studies have revealed a characteristic progression of changes in the hair cells of animals exposed to loud noise. Initially, blebs form on the surface of the hair cells, followed by vesiculation and vacuolization of the smooth endoplasmic reticulum, accumulation of lysosomal granules in the subcuticular region, deformation of the cuticular plate, and finally, cell rupture and lysis (Fig. 66).

Surgery

Patients who have undergone surgery near the inner ear frequently develop vestibular and auditory symptoms during the postoperative period.[5] With *mastoid surgery,* the lateral semicircular canal may be inadvertently opened be-

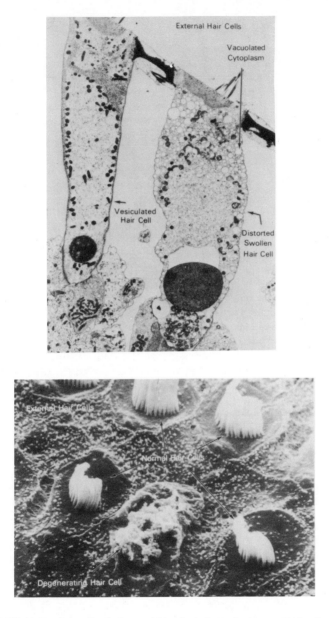

FIGURE 66. Hair cell damage in the cochlea of a guinea pig exposed to loud noise. (A) Transmission electron microscopic section showing vesiculation and vacuolization of the endoplasmic reticulum of the external hair cells; (B) scanning electron micrograph showing a degenerating external hair cell. (From Schuknecht, HF: *Pathology of the Ear.* Harvard University Press, Cambridge, MA, 1974, with permission).

cause of its prominent position in the floor of the mastoid antrum. A perilymph fistula results, and if the membranous labyrinth is torn, the resulting communication between endolymph and perilymph leads to profound unilateral loss of auditory and vestibular function. *Stapedectomy* provides amelioration of severe conductive hearing loss in patients with fixed immobile stapes, but several complications result in disabling vestibular and auditory symptoms. The most important complication, a fistula of the oval window, manifests itself anytime from a few days to months after surgery.[83] Its characteristic symptoms are dysequilibrium, episodic vertigo, and a sensorineural hearing loss that may fluctuate in severity.

OTOSCLEROSIS

Otosclerosis is a disease of the bony labyrinth that usually manifests itself by immobilizing the stapes and thereby producing a conductive hearing loss. Seventy percent of patients with clinical otosclerosis notice hearing loss between the ages of 11 and 30.[84] A positive family history for otosclerosis is reported in approximately 50 percent of cases. Although this disease is considered primarily a disorder of the cochlea, vestibular symptoms and signs are more common than is generally appreciated. Approximately 25 percent of patients with proven otosclerosis complain of episodic vertigo and unsteadiness when walking.[85]

The basic pathologic process of otosclerosis is a resorption of normal bone, often around blood vessels, and its replacement by cellular fibrous connective tissue (Fig. 67).[5] With time, immature basophilic bone is produced in the resorption space; after several cycles of resorption and new bone formation, a mature acidophilic bone with laminated matrix is produced. Areas of predilection for otosclerotic foci include the oval window region, the round window niche, the anterior wall of the internal auditory canal, and within the stapedial footplate. The sensorineural component is perhaps caused by foci of otosclerosis next to the spiral ligament of the cochlea, producing atrophy of the spiral ligament. Otosclerotic foci impinging on the sensory epithelium of the vestibular labyrinth and on the vestibular nerve account for the associated vestibular symptoms.[86]

PAGET'S DISEASE

Paget's disease is a metabolic disorder of bone marked by pronounced osteoclastic resorption of old fully-calcified bone and deposition of new osteoid layers that eventually calcify normally. At times bone resorption resulting from osteoclastic activity is so rapid and extensive that new bone formation lags and the original bone is replaced by fibrous tissue (Fig. 68). The clinical picture varies from the classic one of an enlarged skull, progressive kyphosis, and short stature, to the more common restricted forms confined to the skull, spine, pelvis, and femur.[87] Hearing loss is a common symptom initially described by Paget in his early reports, and subsequently studied in detail by numerous investigators.[5] A progressive combined sensorineural and conductive hearing loss is usually found. The vestibular labyrinth may also be progressively destroyed, resulting in

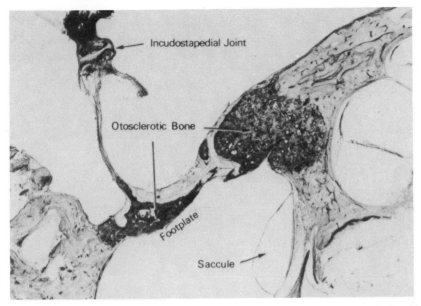

Incudostapedial Joint

Otosclerotic Bone

Footplate

Saccule

FIGURE 67. Histopathologic section showing an otosclerotic lesion involving the bony labyrinth at the anterior margin of the oval window and the entire footplate of the stapes. Patient exhibited a combined conductive-sensorineural hearing loss. (From Schuknecht, HF: *Pathology of the Ear.* Harvard University Press, Cambridge, MA, 1974, with permission).

unsteadiness of gait and, in rare cases, episodic vertigo. In the late stages complete destruction of the bony labyrinth may occur, with invasion of the inner ears by fibrous tissue and new bone formation.

DIABETES MELLITUS

Neurotologic symptoms and signs are common in patients with diabetes mellitus, but convincing evidence does not exist for a disease-specific vestibular disorder.[88] In those diabetic patients with auditory and vestibular dysfunction whose temporal bones and nervous systems have been studied at necropsy, pathologic changes can be explained on the basis of associated vascular disease.[5] Three types of vascular changes occur with diabetes mellitus: (1) endothelial proliferation narrowing the lumens of arterioles, capillaries, and venules; (2) arteriosclerotic narrowing of small arteries and arterioles; and (3) atherosclerotic narrowing of large arteries. These vascular changes may damage the auditory and vestibular systems from the peripheral end organ and eighth nerve to their diffuse CNS connections.

The most common finding in the labyrinth of patients with diabetes mellitus is a PAS-positive thickening of the capillary walls, most prominent in the vascu-

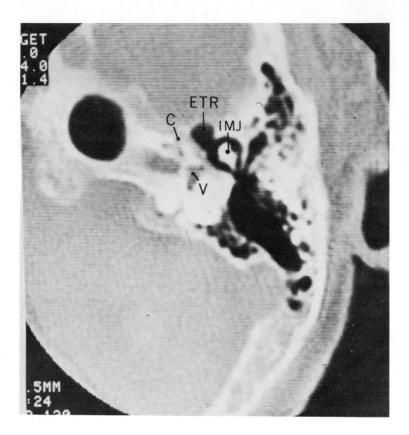

FIGURE 68. C-T scan of the temporal bone illustrating the typical "washed out" appearance in a patient with Paget's disease. C—cochlea, V—vestibule, ETR—epitympanic recess, IMJ—incudomalleal joint. (Courtesy Larry Hoover, M.D., Head and Neck Surgery, UCLA).

lar stria of the cochlea, where it probably accounts for the progressive bilateral high frequency hearing loss characteristic of the disease.[89] Similar changes are found in the vestibular end organs which, along with degeneration of the vestibular nerve and ganglion, could explain the frequent complaints of chronic dysequilibrium and dizziness in diabetic patients.

Sudden onset of hearing loss or vertigo, or both, in patients with diabetes mellitus results from occlusion of the vessels to the labyrinth or the VIII nerve.[88] Cranial nerve mononeuropathy is a well known clinical phenomenon associated with diabetes mellitus, and is most likely due to arteriosclerotic occlusion of arterioles supplying the cranial nerves. Atherosclerosis of large vessels predisposes the patient to transient vertebrobasilar insufficiency and to specific occlusive syndromes such as the lateral medullary syndrome (see Vascular Disorders).

TOXINS

Aminoglycosides

Although all of the aminoglycosides produce auditory and vestibular damage, of the commonly used drugs, streptomycin and gentamicin have their greatest effect on the vestibular end organ, while kanamycin, tobramycin and neomycin cause more damage to the auditory end organ.[5,90] Preliminary studies suggest that two newer aminoglycosides, dibekacin and ribostamycin, are the least ototoxic.[91] Patients receiving aminoglycosides rarely complain of vertigo, but report unsteadiness of gait, particularly at night or in a darkened room. Serial caloric or rotatory examinations can document a progressive bilateral loss of vestibular responsiveness. Hearing loss from aminoglycosides is of the sensorineural type, usually beginning at the high frequencies and progressing to a flat 60 to 70 dB loss across all frequencies. Serial audiograms should be obtained on any patient receiving a prolonged course of aminoglycosides.

The ototoxicity of the aminoglycosides has been convincingly shown to be due to hair cell damage in the inner ear (Fig. 69).[5,92] Unlike penicillin and other common antibiotics, aminoglycosides are concentrated in the perilymph and endolymph, so that the hair cells are exposed to high concentrations of the drugs. Early changes identified by electron microscopy include ballooning of the hair cell surface along with mitochondrial degeneration.[92] Unfortunately, the ototoxicity of aminoglycosides does not correlate with serum drug levels.[93] However, if the total dose is limited to less than 2.0 gm and duration of therapy to less than 10 days, a very low incidence of toxicity can be expected. Since these drugs are eliminated almost exclusively by the kidneys, they should be used with great caution in patients in renal failure.

Salicylates

Patients receiving high-dose salicylate therapy frequently complain of hearing loss, tinnitus, dizziness, loss of balance and, occasionally, vertigo.[94] Sensorineural hearing loss involves all frequencies, and is associated with recruitment, suggesting a cochlear rather than nervous system etiology.[95] The tinnitus is high-pitched and frequently precedes the onset of hearing loss. Both hearing loss and tinnitus invariably occur when the plasma salicylate level approaches 0.35 mg per milliliter. Caloric testing often reveals bilaterally depressed responses consistent with bilateral vestibular end organ damage. All symptoms and signs are rapidly reversible after the cessation of salicylate ingestion (usually within 24 hours). As with aminoglycosides, salicylates are highly concentrated in the perilymph, and preliminary evidence suggests that they interfere with enzymatic activity of the hair cells or the cochlear neurons, or both.[96]

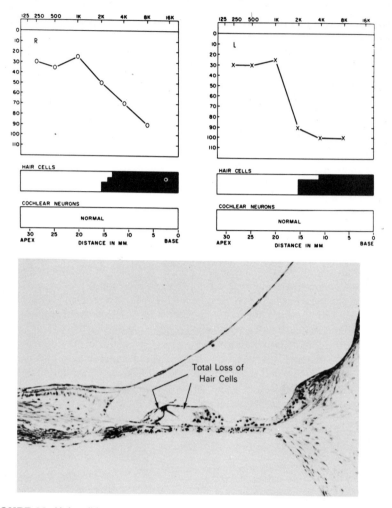

FIGURE 69. Hair cell loss in the cochlea due to kanamycin ototoxicity. (A) Correlation between sensorineural hearing loss and hair cell loss (blackened area) along the cochlea, neurons in the spiral ganglion were normal throughout; (B) histopathologic section of the organ of Corti showing total loss of hair cells in the 8 mm region of the cochlea. (From Schuknecht, HF: *Pathology of the Ear.* Harvard University Press, Cambridge, MA, 1974, with permission).

Other Ototoxic Drugs

The potent diuretics *ethacrynic acid* and *furosemide* have clearly documented ototoxic effects.[5,97] Both drugs produce a rapid onset sensorineural hearing loss that reverses within hours. Animal studies indicate that these so-called "loop inhibiting" diuretics selectively damage the hair cells of the organ of Corti. Combined use of loop inhibiting diuretics and aminoglycoside antibiotics can lead to a profound permanent hearing loss. *Chemotherapeutic anticancer agents,* particularly the alkylating agents, are another group of potent ototoxic drugs.[5] Both the auditory and vestibular labyrinth are affected, with the main pathologic finding being loss of hair cells.

Alcohol

Positional nystagmus and vertigo commonly result from ingestion of alcohol.[98] Within 30 minutes after drinking a moderate amount of alcohol (for example, 100 ml of whiskey) a subject will develop a direction-changing static positional nystagmus often associated with vertigo. The positional nystagmus beats to the right in the right lateral position and to the left in the left lateral position. Nystagmus is not present in the supine position, and is inhibited by fixation. The primary phase of nystagmus reaches its peak in about two hours at approximately the time of peak blood alcohol level (0.1 percent for the above example). Four to five hours after alcohol ingestion, when the blood alcohol level is below 0.01 percent, positional nystagmus is still present, but now is right-beating in the left lateral position and left-beating in the right lateral position (secondary phase). The positional nystagmus can last up to 12 hours, at which time alcohol cannot be detected in the blood.

Alcohol positional nystagmus may be due to a variable rate of diffusion of alcohol into the cupula and the surrounding endolymph.[99] In the primary phase, alcohol rapidly diffuses into the base of the cupula because of the latter's proximity to blood capillaries, while it slowly diffuses into the endolymph. The cupula then has a lower specific gravity than the endolymph, and acts as a gravity sensing organ, maintaining a slight deflection as long as the position is held. After approximately three hours, the endolymph and cupula have approximately the same alcohol concentration, and the positional nystagmus disappears. As the blood alcohol level falls the reverse situation occurs, with the cupula being heavier than the surrounding endolymph, and the secondary phase of positional nystagmus occurs.

BELL'S PALSY

Bell's palsy is a cranial neuropathy of unknown cause usually limited to the facial nerve. However, some patients complain of associated vestibular and auditory symptoms, and careful vestibular and auditory function testing in such patients often reveals objective evidence of VIII nerve involvement.[100] Since a similar combined VII and VIII nerve involvement occurs with a known viral disorder, herpes zoster oticus, and since serologic evidence of viral infection is commonly found in patients with Bell's palsy, several investigators have speculated that Bell's palsy is a viral mononeuritis multiplex.[101,102,103]

MULTIPLE SCLEROSIS

Multiple sclerosis is a CNS demyelinating disease of unknown cause, with onset usually in the third and fourth decades of life. Vertigo is the initial symptom in 5 to 15 percent of cases, and is reported at some time during the course of the disease in approximately 50 percent of patients.[104,105] Hearing loss rarely occurs initially but approximately 10 percent of patients will eventually develop some detectable hearing loss (usually in the later stages).[106] The key to the diagnosis is the finding of disseminated signs of CNS dysfunction manifested in an alternately remitting and exacerbating course. No specific laboratory test for multiple sclerosis exists, but spinal fluid gamma globulin is elevated in 80 to 90 percent of patients at some time in the course of the disease.

CERVICAL VERTIGO

Unilateral interruption of the neck proprioceptive afferents in normal human subjects by injection of a local anesthetic near the upper cervical joints results in vertigo and ataxia.[107] The subjects report a sensation of falling or tilting toward the side of injection, and when walking they deviate toward the injected side. Although animals consistently develop spontaneous nystagmus after unilateral cervical anesthesia, human subjects have not done so despite prominent vertigo and ataxia. This may be due either to a species specificity, or to some difficulty with injecting local anesthetics near the upper cervical vertebrae in humans. Patients with unilateral cervicobrachial radiculoneuritis occasionally develop vertigo and nystagmus during the acute phase of the disorder.[108] Similarly, patients who undergo unilateral sectioning of the upper cervical sensory roots for removal of a tumor may develop vertigo and nystagmus during the first few postoperative days.

A perplexing problem because of the frequency of occurrence and the medicolegal ramifications is the role of soft tissue injuries of the neck (whiplash injuries) in producing vertigo and dysequilibrium. The type of dizziness is often ill-defined, but vertigo is occasionally described. In many instances the dizziness lasts for months or years after the injury, although it usually disappears as swelling and pain subside. From the known anatomic substrate for neck-vestibular interaction (see Chapter 3), it is unlikely that lesions involving only soft tissues of the neck could produce vertigo and dysequilibrium. The major neck afferent input to the vestibular nuclei arises in the paravertebral joints and capsules, with a relatively minor input from the paravertebral muscles. The skin and superficial muscles do not provide any input to the vestibular nuclei. In addition, the relative contribution of neck afferent input to the vestibular nuclei is small compared with direct labyrinthine and visual signals transmitted via the cerebellum. Lesions involving the neck afferents in primates are rapidly compensated for, and therefore prolonged dizziness after neck injuries of any type is difficult to explain on the basis of damage to the neck afferent input to the vestibular nuclei.[9,107]

REFERENCES

1. GOODHILL, V: *Ear Diseases, Deafness and Dizziness.* Harper and Row, Hagerstown, Maryland, 1979.
2. HENDERSON, FW, COLLIER, AM, SANYAL, MA, ET AL: *A longitudinal study of respiratory viruses and bacteria in the etiology of acute otitis media with effusion.* N Eng J Med 306:1377, 1982.
3. PAPARELLA, M, BRADY, D, AND HOEL, R: *Sensorineural hearing loss in chronic otitis media and mastoiditis.* Trans Am Acad Ophthal Otolaryngol 74:108, 1970.
4. PAPARELLA, M, ODA, M, HIRAIDE, F, AND BRADY, D: *Pathology of sensorineural hearing loss in otitis media.* Ann Otol Rhinol Laryngol 81:632, 1972.
5. SCHUKNECHT, HF: *Pathology of the Ear.* Harvard Univ Press, Cambridge, MA, 1974.
6. CHANDLER, J: *Malignant external otitis.* Laryngoscope 78:1257, 1968.
7. FADAN, A: *Neurological sequela of malignant external otitis.* Arch Neurol 32:204, 1975.
8. SCHUKNECHT, H, KIMURA, R, AND NAUFAL, P: *The pathology of sudden deafness.* Acta Otolaryngol 76:75, 1973.
9. BALOH, RW, AND HONRUBIA, V: *Clinical Neurophysiology of the Vestibular System.* FA Davis Co, Philadelphia, 1979.
10. HART, C: *Vestibular paralysis of sudden onset and probable viral etiology.* Ann Otol Rhinol Laryngol 74:33, 1965.
11. ADOUR, KK, SPRAGUE, MA, AND HILSINGER, RL: *Vestibular vertigo. A form of polyneuritis.* JAMA 246:1564, 1981.
12. SCHUKNECHT, HF, AND KITAMUHA, K: *Vestibular neuritis.* Ann Otol Rhinol Otolaryngol 90(suppl. 78):1, 1981.
13. SANDO, I, HARADA, T, LOEHR, A, AND SOBEL, JH: *Sudden deafness. Histopathologic correlation in temporal bone.* Ann Otol Rhinol Otolaryngol 86:269, 1977.
14. HEATHFIELD, G, AND MEE, A: *Diagnosis of Ramsay Hunt syndrome.* Br Med J 1:343, 1978.
15. ZAJTCHUK, J, MATZ, G, AND LINDSAY, J: *Temporal bone pathology in herpes oticus.* Ann Otol Rhinol Laryngol 81:331, 1972.
16. MORRISON, AW: *Late syphilis.* In: *Management of Sensorineural Deafness.* Butterworth, Boston, 1975.
17. WILLIAMS, D, AND WILSON, TG: *The diagnosis of the major and minor syndromes of basilar insufficiency.* Brain 85:741, 1962.
18. FISHER, CM: *Vertigo in cerebrovascular disease.* Arch Otolaryngol 85:855, 1960.
19. FIELDS, WS: *Arteriography in the differential diagnosis of vertigo.* Arch Otolaryngol 85:111, 1967.

20. NARITOMI, H, SAKAI, F, AND MEYER, JS: *Pathogenesis of transient ischemic attacks within the vertebrobasilar arterial system.* Arch Neurol 36:121, 1979.

21. BICKERSTAFF, ER: *Basilar artery migraine.* Lancet 1:15, 1961.

22. EVIATAR, L: *Vestibular testing in basilar artery migraine.* Ann Neurol 9:126, 1981.

23. BASSER, LS: *Benign paroxysmal vertigo of childhood.* Brain 87:141, 1964.

24. EEG-OLOFSSON, O, ODKVIST, L, LINDSKOG, V, AND ANDERSON, B: *Benign paroxysmal vertigo in childhood.* Acta Otolaryngol 93:282, 1982.

25. WATSON, P, STEELE, JC: *Paroxysmal dysequilibrium in the migraine syndrome of childhood.* Arch Otolaryngol 99:177, 1974.

26. POLUS, K: *The problem of vascular deafness.* Laryngoscope 82:24, 1972.

27. COGAN, DG: *Syndrome of nonsyphilitic interstitial keratitis and vestibuloauditory symptoms.* Arch Ophthalmol 33:144, 1945.

28. FISHER, E, AND HELLSTROM, H: *Cogan's syndrome and systemic vascular disease: Analysis of pathologic features with reference to its relationship to thromboangitis obliterans* (Buerger). Arch Path 75:572, 1961.

29. SMITH, JL: *Cogan's syndrome.* Laryngoscope 80:121, 1970.

30. WOLFF, D, ET AL: *The pathology of Cogan's syndrome causing profound deafness.* Ann Otol Rhinol Laryngol 74:507, 1965.

31. FISHER, CM, KARNES, WE, AND KUBIK, CS: *Lateral medullary infarction—the pattern of vascular occlusion.* J Neuropath Exp Neurol 20:323, 1961.

32. BJERNER, K, AND SILFVERSKIOLD, BP: *Lateropulsion and imbalance in Wallenberg's syndrome.* Acta Neurol Scan 44:91, 1968.

33. KOMMERELL, G, AND HOYT, WF: *Lateropulsion of saccadic eye movements. Electro-oculographic studies in a patient with Wallenberg's syndrome.* Arch Neurol 28:313, 1973.

34. ADAMS, R: *Occlusion of the anterior inferior cerebellar artery.* Arch Neurol Psychiat 49:765, 1943.

35. DUNCAN, GW, PARKER, SW, AND FISHER, CM: *Acute cerebellar infarction in the PICA territory.* Arch Neurol 32:364, 1975.

36. SYPERT, GW, AND ALVORD, EC: *Cerebellar infarction.* Arch Neurol 32:357, 1975.

37. PAPARELLA, M, ET AL: *Otological manifestations of leukemia.* Laryngoscope 83:1510, 1973.

38. DINSDALE, HB: *Spontaneous hemorrhage in the posterior fossa: A study of primary cerebellar and pontine hemorrhage with observations on the pathogenesis.* Arch Neurol 10:200, 1964.

39. FREEMAN, RE, ET AL: *Spontaneous intracerebellar hemorrhage. Diagnosis and surgical treatment.* Neurology 23:84, 1973.

40. OTT, KH, ET AL: *Cerebellar hemorrhage. Diagnosis and treatment.* Arch Neurol 31:160, 1974.

41. BRENNEN, RW, AND BERGLAND, RM: *Acute cerebellar hemorrhage. Analysis of clinical findings and outcome in 12 cases.* Neurology 27:527, 1977.

42. TUMARKIN, I: *Otolithic catastrophe: A new syndrome.* Br Med J 2:175, 1936.

43. HALLPIKE, C, AND CAIRNS, H: *Observations on the pathology of Meniere's syndrome.* J Laryngol 53:625, 1938.

44. ALTMAN, F, AND KORNFELD, M: *Histological studies of Meniere's disease.* Ann Otol Rhinol Laryngol 74:915, 1965.

45. BERNSTEIN, J: *Occurrence of episodic vertigo and hearing loss in families.* Ann Otol Rhinol Laryngol 74:1011, 1965.

46. THOMSEN, J, BRETLAN, P, TOS, M, AND JOHNSEN, NJ: *Placebo effect in surgery for Meniere's disease.* Arch Otolaryngol 107:271, 1981.

47. LAWRENCE, M, AND McCABE, B: *Inner ear mechanics and deafness. Special considerations of Meniere's syndrome.* JAMA 171:1927, 1959.

48. ALTMAN, F, AND ZECHNER, G: *The pathology and pathogenesis of endolymphatic hydrops. New investigations.* Arch Klin Exper Ohr-Nas-Kehlkheilk 192:1, 1968.

49. DIX, MR, AND HALLPIKE, CS: *The pathology, symptomatology, and diagnosis of certain disorders of the vestibular system.* Ann Otol Rhinol Laryngol 61:987, 1951.

50. HARRISON, MS, AND OZSAHINOGLU, C: *Positional vertigo.* Arch Otolaryngol 101:675, 1975.

51. BALOH, RW, SAKALA, SM, AND HONRUBIA, V: *Benign paroxysmal positional nystagmus.* Am J Otolaryngol 1:1, 1979.

52. SCHUKNECHT, H: *Cupulolithiasis.* Arch Otolaryngol 90:765, 1969.

53. GACEK, R: *Transection of the posterior ampullary nerve for relief of benign paroxysmal positional vertigo.* Ann Otol Rhinol Laryngol 83:569, 1974.

54. ISHII, T, MURAKAMI, Y, KIMURA, R, AND BALOGH, K: *Electron microscope and histochemical identification of lipofuscin in the human inner ear.* Acta Otolaryngol (Stockh) 64:17, 1967.

55. JOHNSON, L, AND HAWKINS, J: *Sensory and neural degeneration with aging, as seen in microdissections of the human inner ear.* Ann Otol Rhinol Laryngol 81:179, 1972.

56. BRUNER, A, NORRIS, TW: *Age related changes in caloric nystagmus.* Acta Otolaryngol (Stockh) Suppl 282, 1971.

57. MULCH, G, PETERMANN, W: *Influence of age on results of vestibular function test.* Ann Otol Rhinol Laryngol 88 (Suppl 56), 1979.

58. LEWIS, J: *Cancer of the ear: A report of 150 cases.* Laryngoscope 70:551, 1960.

59. SCHUKNECHT, H, ALLAM, A, AND MURAKAMI, Y: *Pathology of secondary malignant tumors of the temporal bone.* Ann Otol Rhinol Laryngol 77:5, 1968.

60. SPECTOR, GJ, ET AL: *Neurologic implications of glomus tumors in the head and neck.* Laryngoscope 85:1387, 1975.

61. GONZALEZ-REVILLA, A: *Differential diagnoses of tumors at the cerebellopontine recess.* Bull Johns Hopkins Hosp 83:187, 1948.

62. MATHEW, GD, FACER, GW, SUH, KW, ET AL: *Symptoms, findings, and methods of diagnosis in patients with acoustic neuroma.* Laryngoscope 88:1893, 1978.

63. YOUNG, D, ELDRIDGE, R, AND GARDNER, W: *Bilateral acoustic neuroma in a large kindred.* JAMA 214:347, 1970.

64. NAGER, G: *Meningiomas Involving the Temporal Bone: Clinical and Pathological Aspects.* Charles C Thomas, Springfield, IL, 1964.

65. KEVILLE, FJ, AND WISE, BL: *Intracranial epidermoid and dermoid tumors.* J Neurosurg 16:564, 1959.

66. NANCE, WE, AND SWEENEY, A: *Genetic factors in deafness in early life.* Otolaryngol Clin North Am 8:19, 1975.

67. KONIGSMARK, BW, AND GORLIN, RJ: *Genetic and Metabolic Deafness.* WB Saunders, Philadelphia, 1976.

68. MONIF, G, HARDY, J, AND SEVER, J: *Studies in congenital rubella, Baltimore 1964–1965. I. Epidemiologic and virologic.* Bull Johns Hopkins Hosp 118:85, 1966.

69. BARR, B, AND LUNDSTROM, R: *Deafness following maternal rubella.* Acta Otolaryngol (Stockh) 53:413, 1961.

70. SCHUKNECHT, HF: *Mondini dysplasia. A clinical and pathological study.* Ann Otol Rhinol Laryngol 89(Suppl. 65):3, 1980.

71. JENSEN, J: *Congenital anomalies of the inner ear.* Radiol Clin North Am 12:473, 1974.

72. MCLAY, K, AND MARAN, A: *Deafness and Klippel-Feil syndrome.* J Laryngol 83:175, 1969.

73. SAEZ, RJ, ONOFRIO, BM, AND YANAGIHARA, T: *Experience with Arnold-Chiari malformation, 1960 to 1970.* J Neurosurg. 45:416, 1976.

74. HEALY, GB: *Hearing loss and vertigo secondary to head injury.* N Eng J Med 306:1029, 1982.

75. DAVEY, LM: *Labyrinthine trauma in head injury.* Conn Med 29:250, 1965.

76. BARBER, H: *Positional nystagmus especially after head injury.* Laryngoscope 74:891, 1964.

77. SCHUKNECHT, H, AND DAVISON, R: *Deafness and vertigo from head injury.* Arch Otolaryngol 63:513, 1956.

78. IGASRASHI, M, SCHUKNECHT, H, AND MYERS, E: *Cochlear pathology in humans with stimulation deafness.* J Laryngol 78:115, 1964.

79. GOODHILL, V: *Leaking labyrinth, deafness, tinnitus and dizziness.* Ann Otol Rhinol Laryngol 90:99, 1981.

80. JAFFE, BF: *Vertigo following air travel.* N Eng J Med 301:1385, 1979.

81. COOPER, JC, AND OWEN, JH: *Audiologic profile of noise-induced hearing loss.* Arch Otolaryngol 102:148, 1976.

82. Davis, H, Morgan, C, Hawkins, J, Jr, et al: *Temporary deafness following exposure to loud tones and noise.* Acta Otolaryngol (Suppl) (Stockh) 88:1, 1950.

83. House, H: *The fistula problem in otosclerosis surgery. Laryngoscope* 77:1410, 1967.

84. Larsson, A: *Otosclerosis: A genetic and clinical study.* Acta Otolaryngol (Suppl) (Stockh) 154:6, 1960.

85. Thomas, JE, Cody, DTR: *Neurologic perspectives of otosclerosis.* Mayo Clin Proc 56:17, 1981.

86. Sando, I, et al: *Vestibular pathology in otosclerosis temporal bone histopathological report.* Laryngoscope 84:593, 1974.

87. Davies, D: *Paget's disease of the temporal bone: A clinical and histopathologic survey.* Acta Otolaryngol (Suppl) (Stockh) 242:7, 1968.

88. Jorgensen, M, and Buch, N: *Studies on inner-ear function and cranial nerves in diabetics.* Acta Otolaryngol (Stockh) 53:350, 1961.

89. Jorgensen, M: *The inner ear in diabetes mellitus.* Arch Otolaryngol 74:373, 1961.

90. Wersall, J, and Lundquist, PG: *Ototoxic drugs.* In Herxheimer, A (ed): *Drugs and Sensory Function.* Little, Brown, and Co, Boston, MA, 1968.

91. Sato, K: *Histopathological study on the vestibular toxicity of six aminoglycoside antibiotics.* Drugs Exptl Clin Res 8:259, 1982.

92. Lundquist, P, and Wersall, J: *The ototoxic effect of gentamicin: An electron microscopical study.* In: *Gentamicin First International Symposium,* Paris, 1967.

93. Fee, WE: *Aminoglycoside ototoxicity in the human.* Laryngoscope 90 (Suppl) 24:1, 1980.

94. Myers, E, Bernstein, J, and Fostiropolous, G: *Salicylate ototoxicity. A clinical study.* N Eng J Med 273:587, 1965.

95. McCabe, P, and Dey, F: *The effect of aspirin upon auditory sensitivity.* Ann Otol Rhinol Laryngol 74:312, 1965.

96. Silverstein, H, Bernstein, J, and Davies, D: *Salicylate ototoxicity. A biochemical and electrophysiological study.* Ann Otol Rhinol Laryngol 76:118, 1967.

97. Mathog, RH, Thomas, WG, and Hudson, WR: *Ototoxicity of new and potent diuretics.* Arch Otolaryngol 92:7, 1970.

98. Aschan, G, and Bergstedt, M: *Positional alcoholic nystagmus (PAN) in man following repeated alcohol doses.* Acta Otolaryngol (Suppl) (Stockh) 330:15, 1975.

99. Money, KE, and Myles, WS: *Heavy water nystagmus and effects of alcohol.* Nature 247:404, 1974.

100. Rauchbach, E, and Stroud, MH: *Vestibular involvement in Bell's palsy.* Laryngoscope 85:1396, 1975.

101. ADOUR, KK, BYL, F, HILSINGER, R, ET AL: *The true nature of Bell's palsy: Analysis of 1,000 consecutive patients.* Laryngoscope 80:787, 1978.

102. DJUPESLAND, G, BERDAL, P, JOHANNESSEN, TA, ET AL: *Viral infection as a cause of acute peripheral facial palsy.* Arch Otolaryngol 102:403, 1976.

103. SANDSTEDT, P, HYDEN, D, AND ODKVIST, L: *Bell's palsy—Part of a polyneuropathy?* Acta Neurol Scand 64:66, 1981.

104. MCALPINE, D, LUMSDEN, CE, AND ACHESON, ED: *Multiple sclerosis. A reappraisal.* Churchill Livingstone, Edinburgh and London, 1972.

105. KURTZE, JF, BEEBE, GW, NAGLER, B, ET AL: *Studies on the natural history of multiple sclerosis: Clinical and laboratory findings at first diagnosis.* Acta Neurol Scand 48:19, 1972.

106. NOFFSINGER, D, ET AL: *Auditory and vestibular aberrations in multiple sclerosis.* Acta Otolaryngol (Suppl) (Stockh) 303:7, 1972.

107. DEJONG, PTVM, ET AL: *Ataxia and nystagmus induced by injection of local anesthetics in the neck.* Ann Neurol 1:240, 1977.108.

108. BIEMOND, A, AND DEJONG, JMBV: *On cervical nystagmus and related disorders.* Brain 92:437, 1969.

10

PROTOCOLS FOR DIAGNOSIS AND MANAGEMENT OF COMMON NEUROTOLOGIC DISORDERS

ACUTE OTITIS MEDIA

Symptoms —Rapid onset of ear pain and pressure, hearing loss.

Signs —Inflamed tympanic membrane, fluid or pus in middle ear, or both.

Laboratory —Positive cultures (spontaneous otorrhea, myringotomy or nasopharynx). Audiometry—conductive hearing loss, flat tympanogram.

Management— Initial empiric antibiotic therapy—Ampicillin.[1,2] Revised antibiotic therapy based on culture and sensitivity tests.

CHRONIC OTOMASTOIDITIS

Symptoms —Chronic otorrhea and hearing loss.

Signs —Pus in external canal, perforation of tympanic membrane (particularly in pars flaccida region) (see Figs. 2 and 3), annular bone erosion, cholesteatoma or granuloma may be visible in the epitympanic region of the middle ear.

Laboratory —Audiometry—conductive hearing loss, restricted or flat tympanogram, absent stapedius reflex. Radiology— nonpneumatized or poorly pneumatized mastoid, haziness of air spaces, bony erosion from cholesteatoma (see Fig. 48). Positive cultures of chronic otorrhea.

Management— Combined medical-surgical. Antibiotics based on culture and sensitivity tests. Surgical removal of granuloma or cholesteatoma combined with mastoidectomy, tympanoplasty, and ossiculoplasty as necessary.[1]

BONY FISTULA OF HORIZONTAL SEMICIRCULAR CANAL
Symptoms —Episodic vertigo induced by cough or sneeze.

Signs —Positive fistula test—brief episodes (10–20 seconds) of vertigo and nystagmus induced by changing pressure in external canal with pneumatic bulb.

Laboratory —Radiology—erosion of bony wall of horizontal canal (see Fig. 48), other signs of chronic otomastoiditis.

Management— Microsurgical removal of the lesion and closure with either perichondrium or fascia.[3]

BACTERIAL LABYRINTHITIS
Symptoms —Acute onset deafness, vertigo, nausea and vomiting.

Signs —Unilateral absent hearing, spontaneous nystagmus, unsteady gait.

Laboratory —Audiometry—profound unilateral (occasionally bilateral) sensorineural hearing loss. ENG—spontaneous nystagmus most prominent with eyes closed or opened in darkness, absent response to caloric stimulation on side of hearing loss. Positive cultures—either pus from middle ear (acute otitis media) or infected cerebral spinal fluid (meningitis).

Management— Antibiotics based on culture and sensitivity tests; symptomatic treatment of vertigo (see Chapter 12).

MALIGNANT EXTERNAL OTITIS
Symptoms —Subacute onset of otorrhea, hearing loss, pain, facial weakness.

Signs —Pus in external canal, ipsilateral hearing loss, and facial paralysis.

Laboratory —Evidence of systemic illness (usually diabetes mellitus). Audiometry—conductive or combined conductive-sensorineural hearing loss. Radiology—increased air cell density and trabecular erosion of mastoid. Cultures positive for Pseudomonas.

Management— Combined medical-surgical. Antibiotics based on cultures and sensitivity tests (usually carbenicillin and gentamicin).[4,5] Extensive mastoid surgery often required.

VIRAL LABYRINTHITIS
Symptoms —Acute onset hearing loss, tinnitus, vertigo, nausea, and vomiting.

Signs —Unilateral hearing loss, spontaneous nystagmus, unsteady gait.

Laboratory —Audiometry—unilateral sensorineural hearing loss, recruitment, normal BAER, and stapedius reflex. ENG—spontaneous nystagmus most prominent with eyes closed or opened in darkness, vestibular paresis on bithermal caloric test.

Management— Symptomatic treatment of vertigo (see Chapter 12).

VESTIBULAR NEURITIS
Symptoms —Acute onset vertigo, nausea and vomiting.

Signs —Spontaneous nystagmus and mild gait unsteadiness (transient).

Laboratory —Audiometry—normal. ENG—spontaneous nystagmus most prominent with eyes closed or opened in darkness, vestibular paresis on bithermal caloric test.

Management— Symptomatic treatment of vertigo (see Chapter 12).

ACOUSTIC NEURITIS
Symptoms —Acute onset tinnitus and hearing loss.

Signs —Unilateral hearing loss.

Laboratory —Audiometry—unilateral sensorineural hearing loss, abnormal BAER or stapedius reflex, or both. Radiology—normal.

Management— Close observation with reassurance.

HERPES ZOSTER OTICUS
Symptoms —Subacute onset of deep burning pain in ear, facial weakness, vertigo, hearing loss.

Signs —Vesicles in external auditory canal (see Fig. 51), unilateral facial paralysis, spontaneous nystagmus (disappears in a few days), unilateral hearing loss.

Laboratory —Culture herpes zoster from vesicle fluid. Audiometry—sensorineural hearing loss, abnormal BAER or stapedius reflex, or both. ENG—spontaneous nystagmus most prominent with eyes closed or opened in darkness, vestibular paresis on bithermal caloric test.

Management— Symptomatic treatment of vertigo (see Chapter 12). Some otologists advocate decompression of the facial nerve during the acute phase. Facial nerve reconstruction surgery or crossover anastomosis to spinal accessory nerve, hypoglossal nerve, or branches of the facial nerve on the opposite side if function does not return.[1]

SYPHILITIC LABYRINTHITIS
Symptoms —Fluctuating but progressive hearing loss, tinnitus and vertigo.

Signs —Interstitial keratitis (see Fig. 52), other manifestations of congenital syphilis (Hutchinson's teeth, saddle nose, frontal bossing, rhagades). Bilateral hearing loss, spontaneous nystagmus (transient).

Laboratory —VDRL positive (75 percent cases). FTA-ABS positive (95–100 percent cases). Audiometry—bilateral sensorineural hearing loss, recruitment present early in course. ENG—spontaneous nystagmus with eyes closed or opened in darkness, bilateral decreased caloric responses.

Management— High dose penicillin (20 million units per day IV × 10–14 days). Steroids (prednisone, 100 mg per day × 10–14 days, maintenance dose if necessary).[6,7]

VERTEBRAL BASILAR INSUFFICIENCY

Symptoms —Episodic vertigo in association with visual hallucinations, visual loss, weakness, drop attacks, visceral sensations, diplopia, headache, dysarthria, ataxia.

Signs —Neurologic examination usually normal, may be signs of prior brainstem or cerebellar infarction, or both.

Laboratory —CT scan—normal. Angiography—often poor correlation between angiographic and clinical findings (see Fig. 55).

Management— Antiplatelet drugs (aspirin 660 mg BID);[8] anticoagulation with heparin for incapacitating, progressing symptoms and signs only[9] (begin heparin 5,000 units I.V. bolus followed by continuous infusion of 1,000 units per hour. Dose is then titrated to keep the partial thromboplastin time at approximately 2½ times control. After 3–4 days warfarin is begun with an oral dose of 15 mg. The daily dose is adjusted (5–15 mg) until the prothrombin time is approximately twice the control value. Heparin is then discontinued).

LATERAL MEDULLARY INFARCTION (WALLENBERG'S SYNDROME)

Symptoms —Acute onset of vertigo, nausea, vomiting, imbalance, incoordination, hiccuping, facial pain, diplopia, dysphagia, dysphonia.

Signs —(1) Ipsilateral Horner's syndrome, (2) ipsilateral loss of pain and temperature sensation on face, (3) ipsilateral paralysis of the palate, pharynx and larynx, (4) ipsilateral dysmetria, dysrhythmia and dysdiadochokinesia, (5) contralateral loss of pain and temperature sensation on body, and (6) spontaneous nystagmus.

Laboratory —CT scan usually normal, high resolution scan may show wedge of infarction in dorsolateral medulla and cerebellum. Angiography—occlusion of ipsilateral vertebral artery in most cases. ENG—spontaneous nystagmus may change direction with loss of fixation, lateropulsion of voluntary saccades, ipsilateral vestibular paresis to caloric stimulation.

Management— Symptomatic treatment of vertigo (see Chapter 12). Antiplatelet drugs (aspirin 660 mg, BID) to prevent future thrombotic episodes.

LATERAL PONTOMEDULLARY INFARCTION

Symptoms —Acute onset of vertigo, nausea and vomiting, hearing loss, tinnitus, facial paralysis, imbalance, and incoordination.

Signs —(1) Ipsilateral hearing loss, (2) ipsilateral loss of pain and temperature sensation on face, (3) ipsilateral dysmetria, dysrhythmia and dysdiadochokinesia, (4) ipsilateral facial weakness, (5) contralateral loss of pain and temperature sensation on body, and (6) spontaneous nystagmus.

Laboratory —CT scan—usually normal, high resolution scan may show wedge of infarction in dorsolateral pontomedullary region and cerebellum. Angiography—occlusion of ipsilateral vertebral artery in some cases. Audiometry—profound unilateral sensorineural deafness. ENG—spontaneous nystagmus that increases with loss of fixation, unilateral loss of caloric responses.

Management— Symptomatic treatment of vertigo (see Chapter 12). Antiplatelet drugs (aspirin 660 mg, BID) to prevent future thrombotic episodes.

CEREBELLAR INFARCTION

Symptoms —Acute onset vertigo, nausea, and vomiting associated with severe imbalance and incoordination.

Signs —Spontaneous or gaze-evoked nystagmus, truncal ataxia, dysrhythmia, and dysmetria of extremities.

Laboratory —CT scan—hypodense lesion of dorsolateral cerebellum (see Fig. 57) may be evidence of distortion of 4th ventricle with brainstem compression. ENG—spontaneous nystagmus changes direction with change in gaze, dysmetria of voluntary saccades, impaired smooth pursuit, and optokinetic nystagmus.

Management— Symptomatic treatment of vertigo (see Chapter 12). Close observation—may require surgical decompression if massive edema occurs.[10]

CEREBELLAR HEMORRHAGE

Symptoms —Acute onset vertigo, nausea and vomiting associated with headache and inability to stand.

Signs —(1) Spontaneous or gaze-evoked nystagmus, (2) nuchal rigidity, (3) facial paralysis, (4) gaze paralysis, (5) marked truncal ataxia, (6) dysrhythmia and dysmetria of extremities, and (7) bilateral small but reactive pupils.

Laboratory —CT scan—circumscribed hyperdense lesion in cerebellum (see Fig. 58), distortion of 4th ventricle, hydrocephalus, and brainstem compression common. ENG—spontaneous nystagmus changes direction with change in gaze, dysmetria of voluntary saccades, impaired smooth pursuit, and optokinetic nystagmus.

Management— Surgical decompression usually required.[11]

LABYRINTHINE HEMORRHAGE

Symptoms —Acute onset vertigo, nausea and vomiting, and hearing loss.

Signs —Spontaneous nystagmus, gait unsteadiness, and hearing loss.

Laboratory —Underlying bleeding diathesis—usually leukemia. Audiometry—unilateral sensorineural deafness. ENG— Spontaneous nystagmus increases with loss of fixation, absent caloric response on side of hearing loss.

Management— Symptomatic treatment of vertigo (see Chapter 12). Treat underlying bleeding diathesis.

COGAN'S SYNDROME

Symptoms —Episodic vertigo associated with progressive bilateral hearing loss and tinnitus.

Signs —Interstitial keratitis (see Fig. 52), spontaneous nystagmus, hearing loss.

Laboratory —VDRL and FTA-ABS—negative. Evidence of systemic vasculitis in some cases. Audiometry—unilateral or bilateral sensorineural hearing loss, recruitment present early in disease process, progression to profound bilateral deafness. ENG—spontaneous nystagmus most prominent with eyes closed or eyes opened in darkness, unilateral or bilateral absent caloric response.

Management— High dose steroids—100 mg prednisone per day × 14 days then gradually taper with maintenance dose if required.[12]

BASILAR ARTERY MIGRAINE

Symptoms —Episodic vertigo, tinnitus, imbalance, incoordination, dysarthria, drop attacks, visual hallucinations or visual loss followed by a throbbing occipital headache; typically occurs in adolescent females with family history of migraine.

Signs —Neurologic examination normal between attacks.

Laboratory —EEG may be abnormal—nonspecific.[13] ENG—vestibular paresis or directional, preponderance to caloric stimulation in about one half of cases.[14]

Management— phenobarbital 60–120 mg per day, propranolol 60–120 mg per day.[13]

BENIGN PAROXYSMAL VERTIGO OF CHILDHOOD

Symptoms —Episodic vertigo, imbalance, nausea and vomiting beginning between ages of 2 to 8 years; approximately one half go on to develop classical migraine attacks.

Signs —Neurologic examination normal.

Laboratory —EEG occasionally abnormal—most commonly diffuse slowing. ENG—vestibular paresis or directional preponderance to caloric stimulation common.

Management—Phenobarbital or dimenhydrinate (dose depending on age and severity of symptoms).[15]

MENIERE'S SYNDROME

Symptoms —Fluctuating hearing loss, tinnitus, ear fullness and vertigo; may have sudden falling episodes.

Signs —Spontaneous nystagmus and gait unsteadiness during attacks, hearing loss that increases during attacks.

Laboratory —Audiometry—sensorineural hearing loss that increases during attacks (see Fig. 41), recruitment usually present; BAER and stapedius reflex usually normal. ENG—spontaneous or positional nystagmus most prominent with eyes closed or opened in darkness, vestibular paresis or directional preponderance to caloric stimulation.

Management— Medical—(1) to prevent attacks—sodium restriction + diuretic (1 gm Na^+ per day and hydrochlorothiazide 50 mg per day),[16,17,18] (2) antivertiginous medication during attack (see Chapter 12). Surgical—(1) endolymphatic sac operations—conflicting evidence of efficacy,[19] (2) destructive procedures (labyrinthectomy or intracranial vestibular nerve section), for patients with disabling vertigo and unilateral severe hearing loss who do not respond to medical treatment (see Chapter 12).

BENIGN PAROXYSMAL POSITIONAL VERTIGO

Symptoms —Brief episodes of vertigo (30 seconds) induced by position change.

Signs —Paroxysmal positional nystagmus induced by rapid change from sitting to head-hanging position, fatigues with repeated positioning.

Laboratory —ENG—paroxysmal positional nystagmus, torsional with upward fast component in both eyes; vestibular paresis to caloric stimulation in approximately one third to one half of cases.

Management— Explanation of the nature of the disorder and its good prognosis helps provide relief. Positional exercises (sitting to both lateral positions) to fatigue nystagmus 3–4 times per day (see Chapter 12, Fig. 70). Transection of posterior ampullary nerve for *rare* intractable cases.[20]

PRESBYCUSIS
Symptoms —Slowly progressive, bilateral hearing loss in the elderly.
Signs —Bilateral high frequency hearing loss.
Laboratory —Audiometry—bilateral sensorineural hearing loss, pure tone pattern (see Fig. 41) may be flat, mildly sloping or severely sloping; occasionally conductive component also present.
Management— Amplification specifically designed for the patient's pattern of hearing loss.[1]

GLOMUS TYMPANICUM TUMOR
Symptoms —Pulsatile tinnitus and hearing loss.
Signs —Reddish mass visible behind the tympanic membrane (see Fig. 3C), ipsilateral hearing loss.
Laboratory —Audiometry—conductive hearing loss.
Management— Surgical removal.[1]

ACOUSTIC NEUROMA
Symptoms —Slowly progressive unilateral hearing loss and tinnitus; vertigo infrequent (in about 10–20 percent of cases).
Signs —Unilateral hearing loss, ipsilateral facial weakness and numbness in late stages.
Laboratory —Audiometry—unilateral sensorineural hearing loss, impaired speech discrimination, abnormal tone decay, abnormal stapedius reflex, abnormal BAER (only wave I present, prolonged I–V interval) (see Fig. 46). ENG—ipsilateral vestibular paresis to bithermal caloric stimulation. Radiology—enlarged internal auditory canal on routine x-rays, mass in cerebellopontine angle with routine CT scan, nonfilling of internal auditory canal with air or metrizamide CT scan (see Fig. 61).
Management— Surgical removal via (1) translabyrinthine, (2) suboccipital, or (3) middle fossa approach.[1,21,22] The translabyrinthine approach destroys the labyrinth, but often allows complete removal of the tumor without endangering other nearby neural structures (particularly the VII nerve). With the suboccipital and middle fossa approaches, residual hearing can be saved, since the labyrinth is not destroyed during the surgical procedure. However, these approaches should probably be reserved for large tumors because of the increased incidence of complications, compared with the translabyrinthine approach.[23]

MALFORMATIONS OF INNER EAR

Symptoms —Long-standing bilateral hearing loss, onset rarely is delayed to adulthood.

Signs —Hearing loss plus evidence of associated malformations of the external or middle ear, or both, ophthalmic lesions, CNS lesions, skeletal malformations, renal disease, thyroid disease, and miscellaneous congenital defects. In majority of cases no other signs present, however.

Laboratory —Audiometry—bilateral sensorineural hearing loss with characteristic V-shaped pure tone pattern (see Fig. 41), BAER normal unless profound deafness. ENG—bilateral decreased caloric responses in approximately one-third of cases. Radiology—tomography or CT scan, or both, may document malformed bony labyrinth.

Management— Amplification where serviceable hearing remains.

CONGENITAL RUBELLA

Symptoms —Congenital hearing loss, usually bilateral, occasionally unilateral.

Signs —Hearing loss with associated congenital defects of the eyes, heart, bone marrow, spleen, liver, and skeleton.

Laboratory —Positive cultures (blood and other secretions) and antibodies for rubella during first 2 years of life; if positive after 2 years of age, more likely that the child contracted rubella on his own. Audiometry—bilateral sensorineural hearing loss with flat pure tone pattern, BAER normal, except with profound deafness. Radiology—tomography or CT scan, or both, may show malformed cochlea.

Management— Amplification if serviceable hearing remains.

ARNOLD-CHIARI MALFORMATION

Symptoms —Oscillopsia and gait unsteadiness.

Signs —Spontaneous nystagmus (typically downbeat), lower cranial nerve palsies, gait and extremity ataxia.

Laboratory —ENG—downbeat nystagmus increases on lateral gaze, no change with loss of fixation; impaired smooth pursuit and optokinetic nystagmus, impaired fixation suppression of vestibular nystagmus. Radiology—herniation of cerebellar tonsils into foramen magnum seen on thin (1.5 mm) CT sections or with metrizamide CT scan (see Fig. 63).

Management— Suboccipital decompression of foramen magnum region.[24]

LABYRINTHINE CONCUSSION

Symptoms —Onset of vertigo or hearing loss, or both, after a blow to the head (usually resulting in loss of consciousness), in some cases onset may be delayed for several days.

Signs —Unilateral hearing loss, spontaneous nystagmus, usually normal external canal and tympanic membrane, may be blood or CSF, or both, in external or middle ear if associated temporal bone fracture.

Laboratory —Audiometry—profound unilateral sensorineural hearing loss. ENG—spontaneous nystagmus most prominent with eyes closed or opened in darkness, decreased or absent caloric response on side of hearing loss. Radiology—usually normal, may be associated temporal bone fracture.

Management— Symptomatic treatment of vertigo (see Chapter 12).

RUPTURE OF OVAL OR ROUND WINDOW

Symptoms —Sudden onset of vertigo and hearing loss after extreme exertion, barometric change, head injury or impact noise.

Signs —May be positive fistula sign—vertigo induced by pressure change in external canal.[25]

Laboratory —Audiometry—unilateral sensorineural hearing loss. ENG—spontaneous nystagmus most prominent with eyes closed or eyes opened in darkness, vestibular paresis to caloric stimulation. Radiology—Normal.

Management— Exploration of middle ear and closure of perilymph fistula.[1]

OTITIC BAROTRAUMA

Symptoms —Sudden, severe ear pain during descent from high altitude or during ascent from underwater diving.

Signs —Hyperemia of tympanic membrane, sometimes with fluid in middle ear, hearing loss on same side.

Laboratory —Audiometry—conductive hearing loss, restricted or flat tympanogram.

Management— Usually spontaneously remits within several hours; if hearing loss persists may require exploration of middle ear to rule out labyrinthine window rupture.

NOISE-INDUCED HEARING LOSS

Symptoms —Gradual bilateral hearing loss and tinnitus with long-standing noise exposure, may be temporary threshold shift with brief exposure to intense sound (e.g., rock concert).

Signs —Bilateral high frequency hearing loss.

Laboratory —Audiometry—bilateral sensorineural hearing loss with characteristic notch at 4000 Hz (see Fig. 41).

Management— Remove from exposure to loud noise. Prevention—carefully monitor hearing levels in subjects at risk (e.g., workers in heavy industry).

OTOSCLEROSIS

Symptoms —Slowly progressive hearing loss and tinnitus (unilateral or bilateral), family history of similar hearing loss, vertigo or unsteadiness, or both, in about one fourth of cases.

Signs —Hearing loss, bone conduction greater than air conduction.

Laboratory —Audiometry—conductive hearing loss (unilateral or bilateral) (see Fig. 40), restricted tympanogram, abnormal stapedius reflex, BAER usually normal. ENG—directional preponderance or vestibular paresis to caloric stimulation in about one half of cases. Radiology—otosclerotic involvement of oval window, round window or bony labyrinth on routine x-rays, polytomography or CT sections.

Management— No proven medical treatment. Amplification—treatment of choice in many cases. Surgery—(1) stapes mobilization (stapediolysis) without removal of any part of the stapes is rarely successful, (2) subtotal stapedectomy—footplate is removed, followed by tissue graft seal of oval window and restoration of part of the stapedial arch, (3) total stapedectomy—removal of the entire stapedial arch, followed by substitution of a prosthesis linking the incus to the oval window.[1]

REFERENCES

1. GOODHILL, V: *Ear Diseases, Deafness and Dizziness.* Harper and Row, Hagerstown, Maryland, 1979.
2. QUARNBERG, Y, AND PALVA, T: *Active and conservative treatment of acute otitis media: Prospective studies.* Ann Otol Rhinol Laryngol 89 (Suppl):269, 1980.
3. GACEK, RR: *The surgical management of labyrinthine fistulae in chronic otitis media with cholesteatoma.* Ann Otol Rhinol Laryngol (Suppl)83:10:5, 1974.
4. CHANDLER, JR: *Pathogenesis and treatment of facial paralysis due to malignant external otitis.* Ann Otol Rhinol Laryngol 81:648, 1972.
5. FADAN, A: *Neurological sequela of malignant external otitis.* Arch Neurol 32:204, 1975.
6. PILLSBURY, HC, AND SHEA, JJ: *Luetic hydrops—Diagnosis and therapy.* Laryngoscope 89:1135, 1979.
7. ZOLLER, M, WILSON, WR, AND NADOL, JB: *Treatment of syphilitic hearing loss: Combined penicillin and steroid therapy in 29 patients.* Ann Otol Rhinol Otolaryngol 88:160, 1979.
8. Canadian Cooperative Study Group: *A randomized trial of aspirin and sulfinpyrazone in threatened stroke.* N Eng J Med 299:35, 1978.
9. GENTON, E, BARNETT, HJM, FIELDS, WS, ET AL: *Cerebral ischemia: The role of thrombosis and antithrombotic therapy.* Stroke 8:150, 1977.
10. SYPERT, GW, AND ALVORD, EC: *Cerebellar infarction.* Arch Neurol 32:357, 1975.
11. FREEMAN, RE, ET AL: *Spontaneous intracerebellar hemorrhage. Diagnosis and surgical treatment.* Neurology 23:84, 1973.

12. BICKNELL, JM, AND HOLLAND, JV: *Neurologic manifestations of Cogan syndrome.* Neurology 28:278, 1978.

13. SWANSON, JW, AND VICK, NA: *Basilar artery migraine.* Neurology 28:782, 1978.

14. EVIATAR, L: *Vestibular testing in basilar artery migraine.* Ann Neurol 9:126, 1981.

15. KOENIGSBERGER, MR, CHUTORIAN, AM, GOLD, AP, AND SCHVEY, MS: *Benign paroxysmal vertigo of childhood.* Neurology 20:1108, 1970.

16. KLOCKHOFF, I, AND LINDBLOOM, V: *Meniere's disease and hydrochlorothiazide—A critical analysis of symptoms and therapeutic effects.* Acta Otolaryngol (Stockh) 63:347, 1967.

17. BOLES, R, RICE, DH, HYBELS, R, AND WORK, WP: *Conservative management of Meniere's disease: Furstenberg regimen revisited.* Ann Otol Rhinol Laryngol 84:513, 1975.

18. GLASSCOCK, ME, DAVIS, WE, HUGHES, GB, AND SISMANIS, A: *Medical management of Meniere's disease.* Ann Otol Rhinol Laryngol 90:142, 1981.

19. THOMSEN, J, BRETLAU, P, TOS, M, AND JOHNSEN, NJ: *Placebo effect in surgery for Meniere's disease.* Arch Otolaryngol 107:271, 1981.

20. GACEK, R: *Transection of the posterior ampullary nerve for relief of benign paroxysmal positional vertigo.* Ann Otol Rhinol Laryngol 83:569, 1974.

21. COHEN, NL: *Acoustic neuroma surgery with emphasis on preservation of hearing.* Laryngoscope 89:886, 1979.

22. PALVA, T, AND TROUPP, H: *Recent experience in the surgery of acoustic neurinomas.* Acta Otolaryngol (Suppl) (Stockh) 360:48, 1979.

23. TOS, M, AND THOMSEN, J: *The price of preservation of hearing in acoustic neuroma surgery.* Ann Otol Rhinol Laryngol 91:240, 1982.

24. SAEZ, RJ, ONOFRIO, BM, AND YANAGIHARA, T: *Experience with Arnold-Chiari malformation, 1960-1970.* J Neurosurg 45:416, 1976.

25. DASPIT, CP, CHURCHILL, D, AND LINTHICUM, FH: *Diagnosis of perilymph fistula using ENG and impedance.* Laryngoscope 90:217, 1980.

11

TREATMENT OF TINNITUS

GENERAL CONSIDERATIONS

MASKING TECHNIQUES

DRUGS

ELECTRICAL STIMULATION

SURGERY

GENERAL CONSIDERATIONS

Most patients with tinnitus can be helped by a detailed interview, together with the relevant examination and laboratory investigations, followed by reassurance where this can be given. Often exacerbating factors such as chronic anxiety and depression can be identified. A "vicious cycle" develops whereby the state of mind makes the tinnitus worse and the tinnitus in turn makes the anxiety and depression worse. The patient may become preoccupied with the tinnitus to the exclusion of all else, feeling that the tinnitus makes life not worth living. Some may even contemplate suicide. The elderly are particularly vulnerable to this problem, since they often have less activity to preoccupy their time. Biofeedback techniques sometimes can be effective in relieving stress and anxiety and thus help break the "vicious cycle" of anxiety and tinnitus.[1,2] In the severely depressed patient, supportive psychotherapy and antidepressant drugs can help to improve the quality of life and reduce the effect of the tinnitus. The American Tinnitus Association provides a unique opportunity for patients to meet fellow sufferers, thereby providing group support and keeping patients informed of progress in the field.

In those patients with hearing loss and tinnitus, a hearing aid may not only improve communication, but also amplification of the ambient sound may effectively mask the tinnitus. This mechanism probably explains the frequent observation that removal of cerumen from the external auditory canal improves tinnitus. When the ear wax is removed the patient hears ambient noise normally and is less aware of the tinnitus. When cerumen is attached to the tympanic membrane, tinnitus may result from local mechanical effects on the conduction system. For patients who find their tinnitus most obtrusive when trying to sleep, a bedside FM clock radio tuned between stations can provide an effective masking sound that will switch itself off after the patient falls asleep.

As indicated in Chapter 6, numerous drugs can produce tinnitus. A careful drug history should be taken and a drug-free trial period considered when possible. Some patients notice that caffeine, alcohol, or nicotine exacerbate their tinnitus and experience significant relief when these drugs are discontinued. Occasionally, occult food additives such as the quinine in tonic water and bitter lemon can be identified as the cause of tinnitus.

MASKING TECHNIQUES

Many patients prefer hearing an external noise (a masking sound) to their own tinnitus. The masking sound may be preferable to tinnitus because it can be more easily ignored. If the patient is not profoundly deaf, it is often possible to generate a sound sufficiently loud to make the patient oblivious of his tinnitus. Although the idea of masking with an external sound source dates back to the time of Hippocrates, tinnitus maskers have only recently been developed and evaluated. These devices are small sound generators that can be worn behind the ear, similar to a hearing aid. The band width of the masking noise is tailored to the patient's tinnitus. Hearing amplification and masking can be combined in the same unit, so that patients with significant hearing loss and tinnitus may also be helped by masking.

As a general rule the effectiveness of tinnitus masking is inversely proportional to the loudness of the masking sound required.[3] Thus, the first step in fitting a masking unit is to identify a sound that effectively masks the tinnitus at the lowest sensation level. Tones, or noise bands, covering the patient's usable hearing range are presented, using an ascending series of sound levels separated by intervals of 2 dB to determine the minimum sensation level required to provide complete masking of the tinnitus. In this way the minimum masking level is determined at each frequency, so that the most effective region of the frequency scale is identified.

One dramatic result of tinnitus masking is the production of residual inhibition, that is, a variable duration of suppression of tinnitus after the masking sound is removed. Residual inhibition occurs in most patients, but unfortunately it usually lasts only a brief time. To test for residual inhibition, a masking stimulus is presented at the minimum masking level + 10 dB for one minute, and the patient is asked to describe the tinnitus when the masking sound is turned off.[3] If the masking stimulus is a good match for the tinnitus, most patients (about 75 percent) will report that their tinnitus is either gone or markedly diminished. The tinnitus usually returns gradually to its pretest level in less than a minute.

TABLE 3. Results of a follow-up survey of 380 tinnitus patients who were provided specific recommendations to participate in the masking program at the University of Oregon, Portland[6]

	MASKERS NO. %	HEARING AIDS NO. %	TINNITUS INSTRUMENTS NO. %	TOTALS NO. %
Recommended for trial purchase	204	132	44	380
Purchased device	93 46	91 69	32 73	216 57
Currently wearing device	61 30(66)[a]	68 52(75)	29 66(91)	158 42(73)
Tried device but did not purchase	58 28	17 13	5 11	80 37
Duration wearing unit				
Less than 1 year	37 40	24 26	12 38	73 34
Less than 2 years	43 46	32 35	12 38	87 40
More than 2 years	13 14	35 39	8 24	56 26
Relief				
Total	6 6	2 2	2 16	13 6
Partial	69 74	39 43	22 68	130 60
None	18 19	50 55	5 16	73 34

[a]Numbers in parentheses, percentages for those patients who purchased instruments and are currently wearing them.

Rarely, residual inhibition will last for several hours after one minute of masking. The degree of residual inhibition with this simple one-minute test gives some indication of the efficacy and success of long-term masking.[3]

Follow-up studies to assess the efficacy of tinnitus masking units have produced variable results. In one study only 9 of 34 patients who were considered candidates for masking units reported that they were receiving some form of relief from their tinnitus.[4] In another study only 10 of 31 patients who rented masking units purchased instruments after a 30-day period and only two of these were using their instruments on a regular basis.[5] The most extensive experience with tinnitus maskers has been accumulated by the group at the University of Oregon in Portland.[3,6] The results of a follow-up survey of patients seen at their tinnitus clinic over a 3-year period from 1976 through 1978 is summarized in Table 3.[6] In this period 493 patients were seen at the tinnitus clinic, and of these 380 were advised to be fitted with one of three instruments: a masking device, a hearing aid, or a combined masking device and hearing aid (tinnitus instrument). In those cases where an instrument was not recommended, the tinnitus could not be effectively masked, or patients indicated that the masking sound was not an acceptable substitute for their tinnitus. Of the 380 patients for whom an instrument was recommended, 158, or 42 percent, were still wearing the instrument after a period of time ranging from 1 to 3 years.

Of the 216 patients who actually purchased an instrument, 73 percent were still using them. Of note, 45 percent of the patients reported that they received total or partial relief of their tinnitus when wearing a hearing aid alone without any additional masking. Very few patients (6 percent) obtained complete relief of their tinnitus with any of the devices.

The relatively poor record of the tinnitus masker alone in this initial evaluation period (only 30 percent were still using the device after 1 to 3 years) could at least in part be attributed to the fact that these instruments were relatively broad band units that contained considerable energy. Many patients reported that their tinnitus was masked, but they rejected the device because the noise was objectionable. Newer tinnitus maskers with high-frequency transducers, narrow bands of noise and low output, may improve patient acceptance of these units. Preliminary assessment of the Oregon group's more recent experience indicates that this may indeed be the case.[6] Furthermore, more patients are being fitted with combined masking and amplifying units as these devices are similarly improved. Additional research is needed to determine the relationship between the effectiveness of a masking stimulus and its band width, spectral composition, and intensity level.

DRUGS

Numerous investigators have reported relief of some types of tinnitus with intravenous lidocaine.[7,8,9] The mechanism of action of lidocaine is uncertain, but it probably acts on the central auditory pathways. Tinnitus that accompanies middle ear disease is not affected by lidocaine. Typically, a maximum dose of 2 mg per kg body weight in 1 percent solution is given intravenously over 3 to 4 minutes. In those patients who experience some relief (approximately 60 percent of patients with tinnitus), the relief lasts between 10 and 30 minutes, but occasionally it lasts as long as several days. Although not a practical long term treatment of tinnitus, the experience with lidocaine provides grounds for optimism that a similar drug might be found that would have prolonged bioavailability when given orally.

Because of the known anticonvulsant effect of lidocaine, several anticonvulsants have been tried in the treatment of tinnitus. Most work has been done with carbamazepine, but in spite of some encouraging initial reports, this drug has now been largely abandoned in the routine treatment of subjective tinnitus.[8,9,10] It should be reserved for patients with intractable severe tinnitus who have a dramatic response to intravenous lidocaine. To minimize side effects, the recommended treatment regimen is to begin 100 mg at night, and then add an extra 100 mg daily each week until the patient is taking 200 mg three times a day, at which time the serum concentration is checked and dosage adjusted.[9] Phenytoin, barbiturates, and sodium valproate have also been used with varying success in the treatment of intractable tinnitus.[9] Also, a number of drugs that are chemically allied with lidocaine are being developed and tested. Controlled clinical trials comparing these different drugs with placebos are needed before their role in the management of tinnitus can be determined.

ELECTRICAL STIMULATION

As part of the recent interest in stimulating the ears of deaf patients electrically, it was observed that positive current could evoke a "silence" sensation in patients with tinnitus.[11,12] An electrical current of positive polarity is produced by passing current from an electrode on the round window to an electrode on the earlobe or mastoid. Subsequently, the procedure has been tried in over 100 patients, with hearing impairment varying from profound deafness to near-normal hearing levels. Suppression of tinnitus was totally effective in 60 percent of the patients tested, and tinnitus could be suppressed at current levels that did not affect hearing in those patients with functional hearing. However, this procedure has obvious risks (e.g., potential permanent damage to the labyrinth) that have not been assessed relative to its potential benefit, and it has yet to be compared with other less invasive methods of treatment.

SURGERY

Surgical treatment of tinnitus has been generally disappointing. Even patients who have undergone removal of acoustic neuromas, or successful stapedectomy surgery for otosclerosis, report variable changes in their tinnitus. In a series of 500 patients who had acoustic neuromas removed, 83 percent had tinnitus before surgery, and in 11 percent tinnitus was the initial symptom.[13] A postoperative survey revealed that tinnitus was improved in 40 percent, worse in 50 percent, and unchanged in the remaining 10 percent. In those patients with otosclerosis whose chief complaint is tinnitus, the tinnitus frequently worsens despite a successful stapedectomy, and if the stapedectomy is unsuccessful, the tinnitus often becomes unbearable.[14] For these reasons, stapedectomy should not be offered as treatment for tinnitus in patients with otosclerosis.

Even when a lesion can be localized to the inner ear or cochlear nerve, removing these structures often has little effect on the tinnitus. Apparently, once the tinnitus is initiated it is propagated in the central auditory pathways, and no longer relies on a peripheral generator. A single exception to the generally dismal record of surgical treatment of tinnitus is complete cure of objective tinnitus after surgical correction of a vascular malformation or tumor in the mastoid.

REFERENCES

1. GROSSAN, M: *Treatment of subjective tinnitus with biofeedback.* Ear Nose Throat J 55:22, 1976.
2. HOUSE, JW: *Treatment of severe tinnitus with biofeedback training.* Laryngoscope 88:406, 1978.
3. VERNON, JA, AND MEIKLE, MB: *Tinnitus masking: Unresolved problems.* In *Tinnitus, Ciba Foundation Symposium.* Pitman Books, London, 1981.
4. ROESER, RJ, AND PRICE, DR: *Clinical experience with tinnitus maskers.* Ear Hear 1:63, 1980.

5. ROSE, DE: *Tinnitus maskers: A follow-up.* Ear Hear 1:69, 1980.

6. SCHLEUNING, AJ, JOHNSON, RM, AND VERNON, JA: *Evaluation of a tinnitus masking program: A follow-up study of 598 patients.* Ear Hear 1:71, 1980.

7. MELDING, PS, GOODEY, RJ, AND THORNE, PR: *The use of intravenous lignocaine in the diagnosis and treatment of tinnitus.* J Laryngol Otol 92:115, 1978.

8. SHEA, JJ, AND HARELL, M: *Management of tinnitus aurium with lidocaine and carbamazepine.* Laryngoscope 88:1477, 1978.

9. GOODEY, RJ: *Drugs in the treatment of tinnitus.* In *Tinnitus, Ciba Foundation Symposium.* Pitman Books, London, 1981.

10. MELDING, PS, AND GOODEY, RJ: *The treatment of tinnitus with oral anticonvulsants.* J Laryngol Otol 93:111, 1979.

11. PORTMANN, M, CAZALS, Y, NEGREVERGNE, M, AND ARAN, J-M: *Temporary tinnitus suppression in man through electrical stimulation of the cochlea.* Acta Otolaryngol (Stockh) 87:294, 1979.

12. ARAN, J, AND CAZALS, Y: *Electrical suppression of tinnitus.* In *Tinnitus, Ciba Foundation Symposium.* Pitman Books, London, 1981.

13. HOUSE, JW, AND BRACKMANN, DE: *Tinnitus: Surgical treatment.* In *Tinnitus, Ciba Foundation Symposium.* Pitman Books, London, 1981.

14. GOODHILL, V: *Ear Diseases, Deafness and Dizziness.* Harper and Row, Hagerstown, Maryland, 1979.

12

TREATMENT OF VERTIGO

GENERAL CONSIDERATIONS

ANTIVERTIGINOUS MEDICATIONS
  Mechanism of Action
  Strategy in Treating Episodes of Vertigo
  Prophylaxis of Motion Sickness

EXERCISE AND VESTIBULAR COMPENSATION
  Mechanism of Compensation
  Vestibular Compensation Exercises
  Positional Exercises

SURGERY
  Rationale
  Labyrinthectomy
  Vestibular Neurectomy

GENERAL CONSIDERATIONS

Vertigo is an extremely frightening symptom. Regardless of the cause, the physician must be supportive and reassuring. If the associated fear and anxiety can be alleviated, the symptom is less distressing. Often the patient suspects that he may have a brain tumor or some other life-threatening neurologic disorder. After the history and examination effectively rule out these possibilities, the patient should be told that his condition is not serious in a life-threatening sense, and that he will respond to treatment. During an acute bout of vertigo, the patient should remain still in bed in a darkened, quiet room. An explanation of how head movements and position changes exacerbate the vertigo during this acute

TABLE 4. Dosage and important effects of several commonly used antivertiginous medications

CLASS	DRUG	DOSAGE	SEDATION	ANTIEMETIC	DRYNESS MUCOUS MEMBRANES	EXTRA-PYRAMIDAL SYMPTOMS
Anticholinergic	Scopolamine	0.6 mg orally q.4–6 h. 0.5 mg transdermally q.3 days	+	+	+ + +	–
	Atropine	0.4 mg orally or intramuscularly q.4–6 h.	–	+	+ + +	–
Monoaminergic	Amphetamine	5 or 10 mg orally q.4–6 h.	–	+	+	+
	Ephedrine	25 mg orally q.4–6 h.	–	+	+	–
Antihistamine	Meclizine	25 mg orally q.4–6 h.	+	+	+	–
	Cyclizine	50 mg orally or intramuscularly q.4–6 h. or 100 mg suppository q.8 h.	+	+	+ +	–

Class	Drug	Dosage				
	Dimenhydrinate	50 mg orally or intramuscularly q.4–6 h. or 100 mg suppository q.8 h.	+	+	+	−
Phenothiazine	Promethazine	25 or 50 mg orally or intramuscularly or suppository q.4–6 h.	+ +	+	+ +	+
	Prochlorperazine	5 or 10 mg orally or intramuscularly q.6 h. or 25 mg suppository q.12 h.	+	+ + +	+	+ +
	Chlorpromazine	25 mg orally or intramuscularly q.6 h.	+ + +	+ +	+	+ + +
Benzodiazepine	Diazepam	5 or 10 mg orally, intramuscularly or intravenously q.4–6 h.	+ + +	+	−	−
Butyrophenone	Haloperidol	1.0 or 2.0 mg orally or intramuscularly q.8–12 h.	+ + +	+ +	+	+ +
	Droperidol	2.5 or 5 mg intramuscularly q.12 h.	+ + +	+ +	+	+ +

stage is often useful. Fortunately, the central nervous system has a remarkable ability to compensate for most types of vestibular imbalance, and therefore, regardless of the cause, acute vertigo will usually gradually resolve within a few days.

As the acute vertiginous episode subsides, the sooner rehabilitation is started, the better the outcome will be. Since vertigo is characteristically made worse by head movements, patients typically hold themselves very stiffly when turning and moving about. They also tire easily with physical activity. At this point it is critical that the patient realizes that a gradual return to normal physical activity is vital to his recovery. In order for the nervous system to recalibrate the relationship between visual, proprioceptive, and vestibular signals, it requires repeated head, eye, and body movements. Patients may drift into a state of chronic invalidism if they are unaware of this requirement.

Treatment of vertigo can be divided into two general categories: specific and symptomatic. Specific therapies include, for example, antibiotics for bacterial or syphilitic labyrinthitis, anticoagulants for vertebrobasilar insufficiency, and surgery for an acoustic neuroma. The specific therapies for most common neurotologic disorders are outlined in Chapter 10. Obviously, whenever possible, treatment should be directed at the underlying disorder. In the majority of cases, however, symptomatic treatment is either combined with the specific therapy, or is the only therapy available (for example, with a viral vestibular neuritis).

ANTIVERTIGINOUS MEDICATIONS

The commonly used antivertiginous medications and their dosages are listed in Table 4. It is apparent that many different classes of drugs are used. As a general rule, the usefulness of each of these drugs has been determined by empiric observation, and in any given individual it is difficult to predict which drug or combination of drugs will be most effective. A patient may respond to one drug, but not to others in the same class.

Mechanism of Action

Numerous animal studies have documented that drugs with anticholinergic and monoaminergic activity diminish the excitability of vestibular nucleus neurons.[1,2,3] *Anticholinergic* drugs suppress both the spontaneous firing rate and the response to vestibular nerve stimulation. Iontophoretically applied acetylcholine, methacholine, and carbamylcholine excite neurons in the medial and lateral vestibular nuclei, and this excitation is blocked with atropine. These observations suggest a likely cholinergic transmission from primary to secondary vestibular neurons. In addition, cholinergic neurons in the nearby reticular formation project to the vestibular nuclei. This reticulovestibular pathway enhances activity within the vestibulo-ocular reflex, and possibly in other vestibular reflex systems as well. Another reticulovestibular pathway is *monoaminergic*. This pathway is activated by amphetamine, and has an inhibitory influence on vestibular nuclei activity induced by electrical stimulation of the VIII nerve.[3]

Thus, there are two separate reticulovestibular pathways, an excitatory-cholinergic and an inhibitory-monoaminergic.[4]

Antihistamines have long been used for the treatment of vertigo and the prevention of motion sickness, yet little is known about their mechanism of action.[4,5] Most antihistamines have some anticholinergic activity, and some also enhance sympathetic activity by blocking the reuptake of monoamines at the nerve synaptic terminals. It may well be that the antihistamines most effective in preventing motion sickness are those with the strongest anticholinergic and monoaminergic-enhancing effects. However, unknown effects on other neurotransmitter systems may be equally important in explaining the antivertiginous effects of antihistamines.

Several tranquilizers are effective in suppressing vertigo. *Diazepam* decreases the resting activity of vestibular nuclei neurons, possibly by decreasing another reticular facilitatory system.[6,7] It also affects crossed vestibular and cerebellar-vestibular inhibitory transmission.[8] The *phenothiazine* chlorpromazine, in addition to its well-known dopaminergic blocking effects, also displays weak antihistaminic and anticholinergic actions. Like the anticholinergic drugs, chlorpromazine suppresses the spontaneous firing rate of secondary vestibular neurons, and also decreases the firing of these neurons following stimulation of the vestibular nerve.[7] Prochlorperazine, a derivative of chlorpromazine, is particularly effective in suppressing nausea and vomiting, presumably through direct action on the chemoreceptive trigger zone in the brainstem. The *butyrophenone* tranquilizers droperidol and haloperidol have antivertiginous and antiemetic properties similar to those of the phenothiazines, and also have the same undesirable extrapyramidal side effects.

Strategy in Treating Episodes of Vertigo

The strategy concerning which drug or combination of drugs to use is based on the known effects of each drug (see Table 4), and on the severity and time course of symptoms.

An episode of *prolonged severe vertigo* is one of the most distressing symptoms that one can experience. The patient prefers to lie still with eyes closed in a quiet, dark room. In this setting sedation is desirable, and the tranquilizing medications listed toward the bottom of Table 4 are most useful. Each of these drugs has important side effects, however, and therefore must be used with caution. Parenteral use of diazepam can cause respiratory depression and hypotension, and therefore should only be used in a hospital setting with emergency resuscitation equipment available. If nausea and vomiting are prominent, the antiemetic prochlorperazine can be combined with the antivertiginous medication.

Chronic recurrent vertigo is a different therapeutic problem, since the patient is usually trying to carry on normal activity, and sedation is undesirable. The antihistaminic, monoaminergic, and anticholinergic medications are useful in this setting. Of the antihistamines, promethazine has the most sedating effect, and is therefore useful only in situations in which moderate sedation is desirable. The administration of promethazine and the sympathomimetic ephedrine (25 mg of each) produces less sedation than promethazine alone, and is more effective in relieving associated autonomic symptoms. Meclizine, cyclizine, dimenhydrinate, and scopolamine are particularly effective in treating mild episodes of vertigo. Transdermal application of scopolamine (transdermal scopolamine 0.5 mg absorbed over 3 days) results in fewer side effects than oral use, and is equally effective in suppressing vertigo.

Prophylaxis of Motion Sickness

As a general rule the antivertiginous medications listed in Table 4 are also effective in treating and preventing motion sickness. Scopolamine was one of the first drugs used in the treatment of motion sickness, and it was the first drug that was proven effective in the prophylaxis of motion sickness. In the 1940s controlled drug trials were carried out on military recruits during amphibious training operations, during aviation training programs, and in swing tests.[9] A dose of 0.6 to 0.8 mg of scopolamine protected from 50 to 60 percent of susceptible subjects over a period of at least 8 hours. With the introduction and subsequent general use of antihistaminic drugs (particularly dimenhydrinate), scopolamine was relatively neglected for many years. However, in the past few years scopolamine has made a comeback in the form of transderm scopolamine. With this delivery system scopolamine is gradually released through a microporous polypropylene membrane contained in a patch that is placed on the skin behind the ear. A small dose (0.5 mg) is slowly released and absorbed over a 3-day period. Initial clinical trials indicate that transderm scopolamine is effective in the prophylaxis of motion sickness with minimal side effects (the main side effect being dryness of the mouth).[10,11] To be effective, the patch must be in place several hours before exposure to motion. Whether other antivertiginous drugs administered in this fashion will be effective in the prophylaxis of motion sickness awaits future studies.

Clinical trials of antimotion sickness drugs under controlled laboratory conditions have shown that combinations of drugs are often more effective than any single drug in the prophylaxis of motion sickness.[12,13,14] Combinations that have been particularly effective include scopolamine 0.6 mg—dextroamphetamine 10 mg, promethazine 25 mg—dextroamphetamine 10 mg, and promethazine 25 mg—ephedrine 25 mg. As in the case of treating vertigo, it is difficult to predict, however, which drug or drugs will be most effective in preventing motion sickness in any given subject. There can be great differences in the response of normal volunteers to the same drug or combination of drugs in controlled laboratory experiments, even where identical motion stimuli are used.

EXERCISE AND VESTIBULAR COMPENSATION

Mechanism of Compensation

As indicated in Chapter 3 the labyrinths maintain a tonic rate of firing into the vestibular nuclei, and this tonic activity in turn is passed on to the motor neurons of ocular and skeletal musculature via the vestibulo-ocular and vestibulospinal pathways. Lesions that produce asymmetry of this tonic vestibular activity result in vertigo, nystagmus, and imbalance. Immediately after an acute unilateral peripheral lesion (e.g., a labyrinthectomy) the ipsilateral vestibular nucleus loses its spontaneous activity and becomes unresponsive to ipsilateral rotation. Animal studies have shown that the nervous system compensates for this abnormality in a predictable systematic fashion.[15,16,17] Initially, the tonic activity of the normal contralateral vestibular nucleus is suppressed so that the asymmetry is diminished. Gradually, a new intrinsic activity is generated in the depressed vestibular nuclei, and the nucleus on the damaged side again responds to angular rotation in both directions. The latter results from activity carried in commissural pathways between the vestibular nuclei, so that the remaining intact labyrinth can drive secondary vestibular neurons on both sides.

The origin of the renewed tonic activity in secondary vestibular neurons several days after a labyrinthectomy is unknown.[18] The source is not an increase in tonic input from the healthy side, since afferent activity in Scarpa's ganglion cells on the normal side remains unchanged. If a second labyrinthectomy is performed after complete compensation for the first occurs, the animal again develops signs of acute unilateral vestibular loss with nystagmus toward the previously operated ear (Bechterew phenomenon), as if the first labyrinthectomy had not taken place. Compensation after the second labyrinthectomy is slightly faster than the first, but still requires several days. The most likely sources of tonic input to secondary vestibular neurons after labyrinthectomy are the cerebellum and reticular formation. Both areas have known anatomic connections with vestibular nucleus neurons, and electric stimulation of parts of the cerebellum and reticular formation results in excitation of secondary vestibular neurons.[18]

In 1946 Cooksey and Cawthorne each reported that in man the vestibular compensation process was more rapid and more complete if the patient began exercising as soon as possible after a labyrinthine injury or ablation.[19,20] Subsequent controlled studies in other primates have supported these clinical observations. Baboons whose hind limbs are restrained by a plaster cast after a unilateral vestibular neurectomy show markedly delayed ataxia compensation, compared with control animals who are allowed normal motor exploration after an identical neurectomy.[21] Squirrel monkeys given daily exercises in a motor-driven rotating cage compensate for a unilateral labyrinthectomy faster than control animals given no exercise.[22] Whether vestibular exercises improve compensation for central causes of vertigo is unknown. If key structures involved in the compensation process are involved (e.g., cerebellum and reticular formation), one might expect little benefit from an exercise program. In fact, such lesions probably explain the occasional patient who shows minimal or no compensation after a central vestibular lesion.[23]

Vestibular Compensation Exercises

The Cawthorne-Cooksey vestibular exercises are outlined in Table 5.[24] These exercises were designed to gradually retrain the eye and body musculature to use vision and proprioceptive signals to compensate for the lost vestibular sig-

TABLE 5. Cawthorne-Cooksey Exercises[19]

A. In bed
  1. Eye movements: at first slow, then quick.
     (a) up and down
     (b) from side to side
     (c) focusing on finger moving from 3 feet to 1 foot away from face
  2. Head movements at first slow, then quick. Later with eyes closed.
     (a) bending forwards and backwards
     (b) turning from side to side
B. Sitting
  1. and 2 as above
  3. Shoulder shrugging and circling
  4. Bending forwards and picking up objects from the ground
C. Standing
  1. as A1 and 2 and B3
  2. Changing from sitting to standing position with eyes open and shut
  3. Throwing a small ball from hand to hand (above eye level)
  4. Throwing ball from hand to hand under knee
  5. Change from sitting to standing and turning round in between
D. Moving About
  1. Circle round center person who will throw a large ball
     and to whom it will be returned
  2. Walk across room with eyes open and then closed
  3. Walk up and down slope with eyes open and then closed
  4. Walk up and down steps with eyes open and then closed
  5. Any game involving stooping and stretching and aiming such as
     skittles, bowls or basketball

---

nals. The eye and head movements listed under A are started as soon as possible after the acute vertigo, nausea, and vomiting subside. The exercises under B through D are then gradually introduced as the patient recovers. Three exercise sessions per day for at least 5 minutes are recommended. Cawthorne suggested that the patient should seek out the head positions and movements that cause vertigo, as far as can be tolerated, since the more frequently vertigo is induced, the more quickly compensation occurs. Antivertiginous medications are used regularly during the course of the exercises to make the vertigo more tolerable.

Grouping patients together for their vestibular exercises is ideal, since members of the group encourage each other and beginners are able to witness the progress of longer term members. The rationale for the exercises should be explained to each patient, and each should be given written instructions outlining the exercise regimen (see Table 5). The exercises are usually continued for 1 to 3 months, and during this time the patient is encouraged to return to a normal work schedule and sporting activities as soon as possible.[24]

Positional Exercises

As indicated in Chapter 9, the natural history of benign paroxysmal positional vertigo is spontaneous recovery in weeks or months, although rarely the condition persists for years. Antivertiginous drug therapy has not proven particularly useful for treating the disorder, since the patient would have to be heavily sedated for a large part of the day in order to suppress the severe brief bouts of vertigo. Based on Schuknecht's proposed mechanism for benign paroxysmal positional vertigo (see Degenerative Disorders of the Labyrinth, Chapter 9), Brandt and Daroff[25] proposed a mechanical therapy using repeated induction of the positional vertigo by positional exercises. They speculated that such exercises would promote loosening and ultimate dispersion of the degenerated otolithic material from the cupula of the posterior semicircular canal. They reported that 66 of 67 patients with typical benign paroxysmal positional vertigo experienced complete relief of their vertigo within 3 to 14 days after starting the positional exercises. My experience has been less dramatic, but the exercises have been effective in some cases. However, some patients prefer to avoid the critical position that induces their vertigo even if it would lead to a more rapid resolution of the problem.

For positional exercising the patient sits with eyes closed and tilts laterally to the precipitating position, with the lateral aspect of the occiput resting on the bed to insure that the posterior semicircular canal is stimulated (Fig. 70). The patient remains in this position until the positional vertigo subsides, and then returns to the sitting position for 30 seconds before assuming the opposite head-down position. This sequence of positionings is repeated until the positional vertigo fatigues. The positional exercises are carried out by the patient every 3 hours while awake, and are terminated after two consecutive vertigo-free days.

SURGERY

Rationale

The rationale for ablative surgical treatment of episodic vertigo is that the nervous system is better able to compensate for a unilateral complete loss of vestibular function than for partial loss that fluctuates in degree. The ideal surgical candidate is a patient with unilateral Meniere's disease who has no functional hearing remaining on the damaged side. Surgery should not be considered if the abnormal side is not well defined, or if the nature of the disease process is unclear. Patients will initially have severe vertigo during the immediate postoperative period (because the asymmetry in tonic activity is increased), but with the exercise program outlined in the previous section, most patients can return to normal activity within 1 to 3 months postoperatively. As a general rule, ablative surgical procedures should be avoided in elderly patients because of the difficulty they have in adjusting to the postoperative ataxia. Two types of de-

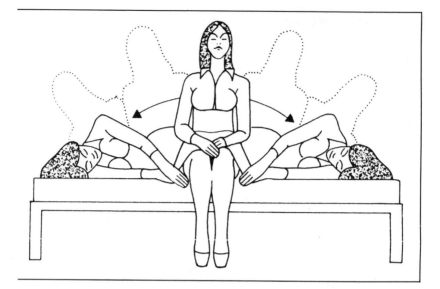

FIGURE 70. Positioning exercises for treatment of benign paroxysmal positional vertigo. See text for details. (From Brandt, T and Daroff, RB: *Physical therapy for benign paroxysmal positional vertigo.* Arch Otolaryngol 106:484, 1980, with permission).

structive surgery are generally in use: labyrinthectomy and vestibular nerve section.[26,27]

Labyrinthectomy

Labyrinthectomy is useful only in those situations where no functional hearing remains on the side to be operated upon. The goal of a labyrinthectomy is to remove the neuroepithelium of the vestibular end organ. Trans-oval-window or trans-round-window exenterations are simple procedures that may be effective, but parts of the neuroepithelium are often left behind, which may lead to a return of episodic vertigo. For total removal of the vestibular neuroepithelium, a translabyrinthine labyrinthectomy is required. With this procedure the surgeon first performs a simple mastoidectomy to outline the three semicircular canals. Next the canals are opened, their neuroepithelium removed, and the dissection is carried into the vestibule, where the remaining neuroepithelium is identified and removed. The operation can be extended at this point to include section of the superior and inferior division of the vestibular nerve in the internal auditory canal. Major complications with this procedure are infrequent, since hearing is not a factor, the subarachnoid space is not violated, and the facial nerve is usually not exposed in areas where it is not covered by a thick sheath. Wound infection is the most common complication.

Vestibular Neurectomy

Vestibular neurectomy offers the possibility of hearing conservation in cases with salvageable residual cochlear function, but the risks of complications are greater. Initially the neurosurgical suboccipital approach to the cerebellopontine angle was used for intracranial section of the vestibular nerve. This is a major surgical procedure with significant morbidity and occasional mortality that is probably unwarranted as a treatment for episodic vertigo. More recently, a safer middle cranial fossa approach to the vestibular nerve has been developed.[26,28] Complications of this procedure include trauma to the facial and cochlear nerves (5 to 10 percent of patients will lose hearing on the side of operation), postoperative cerebrospinal fluid leak, and subdural or epidural hematoma.

REFERENCES

1. YAMAMOTO, C: *Pharmacologic studies of norepinepherine, acteylcholine, and related compounds in Deiter's nucleus and cerebellum.* J Pharmacol Exp Ther 156:39, 1967.

2. JAJU, BP, KIRSTEN, EB, AND WANG, SC: *Effects of belladonna alkaloids on vestibular nucleus of the cat.* Am J Physiol 219:1248, 1970.

3. MATSUOKA, I, DOMINO, EF, AND MORIMOTO, M: *Adrenergic and cholinergic mechanisms of single vestibular neurons in the cat.* Adv Otorhinolaryngol. 19:163, 1973.

4. BROWN, RD, AND WOOD, CD: *Vestibular Pharmacology. Trends in Pharmacological Sciences.* p 150, February 1980.

5. JAJU, BP, AND WANG, SC: *Effects of diphenhydramine and dimenhydrinate on vestibular neuronal activity of cat: A search for the locus of their antimotion sickness action.* J Pharmacol Exp Therap 176:718, 1971.

6. RYU, JH, AND MCCABE, BF: *Effects of diazepam and dimenhydrinate on the resting activity of the vestibular neuron.* Aerospace Medicine 10:1117, 1974.

7. MATSUOKA, I, CHIKAMORI, Y, TAKAORI, S, AND MORIMOTO, M: *Effects of chlorpromazine and diazepam on neuronal activities of the lateral vestibular nucleus in cats.* Arch Otorhinolaryngol 209:89, 1975.

8. STEINER, FA, AND FELIX, D: *Antagonistic effects of GABA and benzodiazepines on vestibular and cerebellar neurons.* Nature 260:346, 1976.

9. BARD, P: *Motion sickness.* In ANDRUS, EC, BRONK, DW, CARDEN, GA, ET AL (EDS): *Advances in Military Medicine.* Little Brown and Co, Boston, 1948.

10. MCCAULEY, ME, ROYAL, JW, SHAW, JE, AND SCHMITT, LG: *Effect of transdermally administered scopolamine in preventing motion sickness.* Aviat Space Environ Med 50:1108, 1979.

11. PRICE, N, SCHMITT, LG, AND SHAW, JE: *Transdermal delivery of scopolamine for prevention of motion-induced nausea in rough seas.* Clin Therap 2:258, 1979.

12. WOOD, CD, AND GRAYBIEL, A: *Evaluation of sixteen antimotion sickness drugs under controlled laboratory conditions.* Aerospace Medicine 39:1342, 1968.
13. WOOD, CD, AND GRAYBIEL, A: *Evaluation of antimotion sickness drugs: A new effective remedy revealed.* Aerospace Medicine 41:932, 1970.
14. GRAYBIEL, A, WOOD, CD, KNEPTON, J, HOCHE, JP, AND PERKINS, GF: *Human assay of antimotion sickness drugs.* Aviat Space Environ Med 46:1107, 1975.
15. PRECHT, W, SHIMAZU, H, AND MARKHAM, CH: *A mechanism of central compensation of vestibular function following hemilabyrinthectomy.* J Neurophysiol 29:996, 1966.
16. McCABE, BF, AND RYU, JH: *Experiments on vestibular compensation.* Laryngoscope 79:1728, 1969.
17. DIERINGER, N, AND PRECHT, W: *Mechanisms for vestibular deficits in the frog.* Exp Brain Res 36:329, 1979.
18. PRECHT, W: *The physiology of the vestibular nuclei.* In KORNHUBER, HH (ED): *Handbook of Sensory Physiology. The Vestibular System, vol VI, part 1.* Springer-Verlag, New York 1974.
19. COOKSEY, FS: *Rehabilitation in vestibular injuries.* Proc Roy Soc Med 39:220, 1945.
20. CAWTHORNE, T: *Vestibular injuries.* Proc Roy Soc Med 39:270, 1945.
21. LACOUR, M, ROLL, JP, AND APPAIX, M: *Modifications and development of spinal reflexes in the alert baboon (papio papio) following a unilateral vestibular neurotomy.* Brain Res 113:255, 1976.
22. IGARASHI, M, LEVY, JK, O-UCHI, T, AND RESCHKE, MF: *Further study of physical exercise and locomotor balance compensation after unilateral labyrinthectomy in squirrel monkeys.* Acta Otolaryngol (Stockh) 92:101, 1981.
23. RUDGE, R: *Physiological basis for enduring vestibular symptoms.* J Neurol Neurosurg Psychiatry 45:126, 1982.
24. DIX, MR: *The rationale and technique of head exercises in the treatment of vertigo.* Acta Otorhinolaryng Belg 33:370, 1979.
25. BRANDT, T, AND DAROFF, RB: *Physical therapy for benign paroxysmal positional vertigo.* Arch Otolaryngol 106:484, 1980.
26. GOODHILL, V: *Ear Diseases, Deafness and Dizziness.* Harper and Row, Hagerstown, Maryland, 1979.
27. FISCH, U: *Surgical treatment of vertigo.* J Laryngol Otol 90:75, 1976.
28. GLASSCOCK, ME, DAVIS, WE, HUGHES, GB, AND JACKSON, CG: *Labyrinthectomy versus middle fossa vestibular nerve section in Meniere's disease.* Ann Otol Rhinol Laryngol 89:318, 1980.

INDEX

A page number in italics indicates an illustration; a *t* following a page number indicates a table.

eighth nerve and, 27–28
fluid dynamics of, 16–18, *17*
fluids of
  chemical composition of, 17
labyrinth and
  development of, 14, *15,* 16
  phylogeny of, 13–14
physiology of, 13–30
receptor organs of, 20, 22–23, *22, 24,*
  25, *25, 26,* 27
Intralabyrinthine hemorrhage, 128–129

KANAMYCIN, ototoxicity and, 149, *150*
Keratinizing squamous epithelium, oto-
  mastoiditis and, 115, *116*
Keratitis, interstitial, syphilitic infections
  and, 120, *122*
Keratoma, in middle ear, 8
Klippel-Feil syndrome, 139

LABYRINTH
  degenerative disorders of, 132–133,
    135
  development of, 14, *15,* 16
  membranous
    rupture of, 17
  phylogeny of, 13–14
Labyrinthine concussion, 142
  management of, 167–168
Labyrinthine hemorrhage, management
  of, 164
Labyrinthine infarction, 126
Labyrinthectomy
  as treatment for vertigo, 186
  nystagmus following
    ENG recordings of, *85*
Labyrinthitis
  bacterial, 117
    management of, 160
  hearing loss and, 68
  syphilitic
    management of, 161–162
    syphilitic infections and, 120–121
  temporal bone in, *118*
  viral, 117, 120
    management of, 160–161
Lateral medullary infarction, management of, 162–163
Lateral pontomedullary infarction, management of, 163

Lateral pontomedullary syndrome, 127
Lateral vestibulospinal tract. *See* Vesti-
  bulospinal tract, lateral.
Lesion(s), neurologic, visual ocular con-
  trol abnormalities and, 93t
Leukemia, intralabyrinthine hemorrhage
  and, 128
Lidocaine, for tinnitus, 174
Light-headedness, presyncopal, vestib-
  ular lesions and, 61

MACULE, of inner ear, 20, 22–23, *22*
Mal de debarquement syndrome, 65
Masking techniques, for treatment of tinnitus, 172–174, 173t
Mastoid antrum, 3
Mastoid surgery, symptoms following,
  144
Meclizine, for treatment of vertigo,
  178t–179t
Medial geniculate body, 53
Medial longitudinal fasciculus (MLF), 33
  nystagmus and, 82
Medial vestibulospinal tract. *See* Vestibulospinal tract, medial.
Meniere's syndrome, 17, 129, 131–132,
  132
  idiopathic
    genetic factors in, 131
  labyrinth in, *132*
  management of, 165
  relapsing hearing loss and, 58
  tinnitus and, 70
  transient dizziness in, 62
Meningioma(s), 137
Meningitis, temporal bone in, *118*
Michel deformity, 139
Middle ear
  anatomy of, 3–11
  cholesteatoma in, 8
  components of, 3
  development of, 4–5, *4*
  eustachian tube and, *4,* 5–7, *6*
  facial nerve and, 9–10, *9*
  keratoma in, 8
  ossicular chain and, 8
  physiology of, 3–11
  temporal bone and, 3
  tympanic cavity and
    boundaries of, 5, *6*

spontaneous, 35–36, 77–78
  causes of
    differentiation of, 78
    congenital, 78
  recording of
    electronystagmography and, 85

PAGET'S disease, 146–147, 148
Parkinson's disease, saccadic reaction
    and, 92
Paroxysmal positional nystagmus. See
    Nystagmus, positional, parox-
    ysmal.
Past pointing, impaired vestibular func-
    tion and, 74, 75
Pathologic nystagmus. See Nystagmus,
    pathologic.
Penicillin, syphilitic labyrinthitis and, 162
Perilymph fistula(ae), 142, 143
Phenobarbital
  in basilar artery migraine, 165
  in benign paroxysmal vertigo of child-
    hood, 165
Phenytoin, for tinnitus, 174
Polypoid granuloma(s), otomastoiditis
    and, 115
Positional nystagmus. See Nystagmus,
    positional.
Posture
  imbalance of
    vestibular lesions and, 62
  vestibular influence on, 43
Prednisone
  in Cogan's syndrome, 164
  syphilitic labyrinthitis and, 162
Presbycusis, 68–69, 133, 135
  audiogram in, 100, 135
  management of, 166
Presyncopal light-headedness, vestibu-
    lar lesions and, 61
Prochlorperazine for treatment of ver-
    tigo, 178t–179t, 181
Promethazine, for treatment of vertigo,
    178t–179t
Propranolol, in basilar artery migraine,
    165
Pure tone studies, for hearing loss, 98,
    99

REBOUND nystagmus. See Nystagmus,
    rebound.

Reflex(es). See also under individual
    names.
  acoustic, 52
    measurement of, 103–104, 104t
    stapedius, 51–52, 52
    Bell's palsy and, 51
Reissner's membrane, 25
Reticulospinal tract, 42
Rhombencephalon, 14
Ribostamycin, ototoxicity and, 149
Rinne test, 97–98
Romberg test, 74, 75
Rotatory testing
  nystagmus induced by, 89
  results of
    interpretation of, 89–90
    technique for, 88–89
Round window, rupture of, management
    of, 168
Rubella
  congenital
    hearing loss with
      management of, 167
    congenital ear malformation and, 138
Russell's hook bundle, 43

SACCADE(S), 91
  reaction time of
    alteration in
      causes of, 92
Saccade dysmetria, 92
Saccule, macule and, 20
Salicylates, ototoxicity and, 149
Scarpa's ganglion, 28
Schwannoma(s)
  facial nerve, 136
  vestibular, 136–137, 137
    hearing loss and, 68
Scopolamine, for treatment of vertigo,
    178t–179t
Shrapnell's membrane, 8
Smooth pursuit, 91
  abnormal, 93
Sodium valproate, for tinnitus, 174
Sound pressure level (SPL), acoustic im-
    pedance and, 101
Speech discrimination test, 99
Speech reception threshold (SRT), 99
Speech studies, in hearing loss, 99
Speech test(s), central auditory,
    107–108